ADVANCED IN APPLIED SCIENCE AND ENGINEERING

COVID-19 PANDEMIC

QUESTIONS, ANSWERS AND HYPOTHESES

ADVANCED IN APPLIED SCIENCE AND ENGINEERING

Additional books and e-books in this series can be found on Nova's website under the Series tab.

ADVANCED IN APPLIED SCIENCE AND ENGINEERING

COVID-19 PANDEMIC

QUESTIONS, ANSWERS AND HYPOTHESES

A. K. HAGHI
EDITOR

nova
Medicine & Health
New York

NOTICE TO THE READER

Library of Congress Cataloging-in-Publication Data

Names: Haghi, A. K., author. Title: COVID-19 pandemic : questions, answers and hypotheses / A.K. Haghi, Professor Emeritus of Engineering Sciences, University of Guilan, Iran. Description: New York : Nova Science Publishers, [2020] | Series: Infectious disease and microbiology | Includes bibliographical references and index. | Summary: "Since the early 2020s, the entire world has been in panic and confusion due to the coronavirus that causes COVID-19. To protect ourselves from the virus, national borders have been closed and people have been ordered to stay home. The world was practically isolated under martial law. The global lockdown caused a total social and economic disruption. After the events that have happened today, we need to be prepared for further changes that will soon affect our lives. This book summarizes the Covid19 pandemic in general, warning us of the dangers it poses beyond the disease. The loss of freedom enjoyed by the western world could be at risk if governments do not moderate authoritarianism and follow the terrible example of countries that do not know or enjoy such freedoms. We save lives but preserve our lifestyle"-- Provided by publisher.
Identifiers: LCCN 2020038601 (print) | LCCN 2020038602 (ebook) | ISBN 9781536185652 (paperback) | ISBN 9781536185935 (adobe pdf) Subjects: LCSH: COVID-19 (Disease) | Epidemics--Social aspects. | Epidemics--Economic aspects. | Quarantine--Social aspects.
Classification: LCC RA644.C67 H34 2020 (print) | LCC RA644.C67 (ebook) | DDC 614.5/92414--dc23
LC record available at https://lccn.loc.gov/2020038601
LC ebook record available at https://lccn.loc.gov/2020038602

Published by Nova Science Publishers, Inc. † New York

CONTENTS

PREFACE

The COVID-19 pandemic is accelerating and the world has not reached the peak of the global outbreak. The number of cases is increasing, but it is still possible to minimize transmission. While the number of deaths appears to have leveled off globally, in reality some countries have made significant progress in reducing the number of deaths, while deaths are still on the rise in other countries. We have been saying for a long time now, including at the early stages of the pandemic that this virus is very dangerous, and we called it many times public enemy number one.

Many scientists were waiting for the arrival of a virus as the cause of COVID-19, what they could not predict was when it would happen. In this volume the history of other pandemics is revised, and what lessons people can draw from them and, perhaps, what they could have avoided are discussed. Learning from the past is key to anticipating a disaster as COVID-19.

In: COVID-19 Pandemic
Editor: A. K. Haghi
ISBN: 978-1-53618-565-2

Chapter 1

COVID-19, HYDROXYCHLOROQUINE, DRUG REPURPOSING AND MATHEMATICS

Francisco Torrens[1,*] and Gloria Castellano[2]
[1]Institut Universitari de Ciència Molecular, Universitat de València, Edifici d'Instituts de Paterna, València, Spain
[2]Departamento de Ciencias Experimentales y Matemáticas, Facultad de Veterinaria y Ciencias Experimentales, Universidad Católica de Valencia San Vicente Mártir, València, Spain

ABSTRACT

This review refers to the *grouting* of glances in relation to a subject. The ideas *are already circulating*, and the task is to enable access. One does not stop seeing his confirmed suspicions when thinking about the situation, *via* the lens of the *state of exception* and a government that limits freedoms in the name of security. Another suggests that the crisis will force people to think of an alternative society, beyond the nation state, and they must *reinvent communism based on trust in people and in science*; i.e., each expert brings water to his own mill, and *uses* the current crisis to confirm the disasters that his theories already predicted or

* Corresponding Author's E-mail: torrens@uv.es.

promote the type of government he prefers. What time of thought do people live in? It seems that the epidemic test everywhere dissolves Reason intrinsic activity and forces the subjects to return to the sad effects common in the Middle Ages. To think expertly about an event, e.g., this, requires time, etc. What is done, in a hurry, is usually to reduce otherness to the same: Confine it in the usual parameters of its own, in orbit of the self, of the known.

Keywords: SARS-CoV2, chloroquine, systemic lupus erythematosus, immunomodulation, malaria, antiviral, new drug

1. INTRODUCTION

Setting the scene: pandemic history, meeting the family, whether people could predict the coronavirus (CoV) pandemic, what lessons we have learned from other pandemics, severe acute respiratory syndrome (SARS) CoV as an agent of emerging and reemerging infection, whether people should be ready for the reemergence of SARS, global shifts in mammalian population trends revealing key predictors of virus spillover risk, the proximal origin of SARS-CoV clade 2 (SARS-CoV-2), an interactive web-based dashboard to track CoV disease 2019 (COVID-19) in real time (RT), COVID-19, globalization, coalition, advocacy for prospective clinical trials (CTs) to test the post-exposure potential of hydroxychloroquine (HCQ) *vs.* COVID-19, drug repurposing for CoV treatment, computational study based on molecular topology (MT), mathematics to explain the measures *vs.* CoV, the curve, why COVID-19 curve is so important, whether a virus can undermine human rights (HRs), answering the right questions for policymakers on COVID-19, building trust while influencing online COVID-19 content in the social media world, ethnicity, COVID-19, an urgent public health (PH) research priority, nowcasting and forecasting the potential domestic and international spread of the SARS-CoV-2 outbreak originating in Wuhan, China, a modelling study, offline, COVID-19, the NHS, *a national scandal*, the novel CoV outbreak, what people know, what they do not,

COVID-19, navigating uncertainties together, COVID-19 being a data science issue, differentiating COVID-19 response strategies, COVID-19, imbalanced host response to SARS-CoV-2 driving development of COVID-19, a multibasic cleavage site in the spike protein of SARS-CoV-2 being essential for infection of human lung cells, and SARS-CoV-2 receptor angiotensin-converting enzyme 2 (ACE2) being an interferon-stimulated gene in human airway epithelial cells, being detected in specific cell subsets across tissues, full-genome evolutionary analysis of the novel CoV (SARS-CoV-2) rejects the hypothesis of emergence as a result of a recent recombination event, pathogenicity, transmissibility of SARS-CoV-2, a quick overview, comparison with other emerging viruses, SARS-CoV-2, COVID-19, the epidemic, the challenges, insights into the recent 2019 novel SARS-CoV-2 in light of past human CoV (HCoV) outbreaks, insight into 2019 novel CoV, an updated interim review, lessons from SARS-CoV and Middle East respiratory syndrome (MERS)-CoV, sex-bias in COVID-19, a meta-analysis and review of sex differences in disease and immunity, COVID-19 evolving in human hosts, COVID-19, a lesson in humility, an opportunity for sagacity, hope, COVID-19, the isolation that has brought people together, an RT dashboard of CTs for COVID-19, COVID-19 as a new virus, but a familiar receptor and cytokine release syndrome, impact of contact tracing on SARS-CoV-2 transmission, what policy makers need to know about COVID-19 protective immunity, isolation, inclusion, key ethical questions for research during COVID-19 pandemic, virtual treatment, *social distancing*, PH messaging, harm reduction in the time of COVID-19, decolonising COVID-19, trained immunity, a tool for reducing susceptibility and severity of SARS-CoV-2 infection, herd immunity, understanding COVID-19, clinical features of patients infected with 2019 novel CoV in Wuhan, China, genomic characterisation and epidemiology of SARS-CoV-2, implications for virus origins and receptor binding, molecular modelling (MM) and docking studies of DTQ, THQ, THY, TQ compounds compared with HCQ targeting receptor-binding domain (RBD) of SARS-CoV-2 drug target towards finding their potential to act as anti-CoV drug-like small molecule, etiology of epidemic outbreaks COVID-19 in Wuhan, Hubei province, Chinese People Republic associated with

SARS-CoV-2 (*Nidovirales, Coronaviridae, Coronavirinae, Betacoronavirus*, subgenus *Sarbecovirus*), lessons of SARS-CoV outbreak, *not touching*, science *vs.* disinformation in *COVID-19* pandemic, ethics, COVID-19, resource allocation, priority-setting, offline, a global health crisis, something far worse, navigating the clean energy transition in COVID-19 crisis, epidemiological, clinical characteristics of 99 cases of SARS-CoV-2 pneumonia in Wuhan, China, a descriptive study, SARS-CoV-2 isolation, rapid sharing from the first patient diagnosed with COVID-19 in Australia, European response to COVID-19, from regulatory emulation to regulatory coordination, CoV infections, more than just the common cold, association of PH interventions with the epidemiology of COVID-19 outbreak in Wuhan, China, choices for the *new normal*, COVID-19, remaking the social contract, COVID-19 putting societies to the test, community participation being crucial in a pandemic, managing disasters amid COVID-19 pandemic, approaches of response to flood disasters, quantifying SARS-CoV-2 transmission suggesting epidemic control with digital contact tracing, senolytics improving physical function, increasing lifespan in old age, estimates of the severity of COVID-19, a model-based analysis COVID-19, death rate being 0.66%, increasing with age, study estimates, understanding CoV, the equitable distribution of COVID-19 therapeutics, vaccines, COVID-19 being neither created nor escaped from a laboratory, COVID-19, the dark side of the promiscuity of life, SARS-CoV-2 origin in light of evolution, what virologists know to date about SARS-CoV-2, COVID-19, teachers, mutation, extinction, university teachers in the digital age, adapting, dying, the university having to be renewed in a virtual environment without losing its essence, educating in times of confinement, the task of renewing a common world, teachers, students, families talking about non-contact education, COVID-19, pandemic of mathematical models, not all data being the same, the importance of context in pandemic information, CoV, ruling out reinfection in cures, being *false positives*, CoV, double warning over antibody (Ab) tests, more cases of reinfected ones raising doubts about immunity, what is happening, alleged reinfected by coronavirus being *false positives*, South Korea (SK) saying, clinical characteristics of the recovered COVID-19 patients with re-detectable positive ribonucleic acid (RNA) test, good practices in the work centres, measures for the prevention of contagions of COVID-19, the arrival of COVID-19 in a context of climate emergency, the consequences of a crisis of crises, gender, COVID-19, advocacy brief, autopsy slowdown hinders quest to determine how coronavirus kills, severe COVID-19, a review of recent progress with a look towards the future, dynamics in a simple evolutionary-epidemiological model for the evolution of an initial asymptomatic infection stage, the airborne lifetime of small speech droplets, their potential importance in SARS-CoV-2 transmission, a novel bat CoV closely related to SARS-CoV-2 containing natural insertions at S1/S2 cleavage site of the spike protein, whether pangolins are the intermediate host of SARS-CoV-2, cross-neutralization of SARS-CoV-2 by a human SARS-CoV monoclonal (m)Ab, whether photography is a lie, lessons from the pandemic, the stress test that is the pandemic surfacing strengths, weaknesses, airway driving pressure, lung stress in acute respiratory distress syndrome (ARDS) patients, driving pressure, survival in ARDS, lactic acidosis, an update, extracorporeal membrane oxygenation for severe ARDS, whether trauma or growth after a natural disaster, the mediating role of rumination processes, whether trauma or personal growth, possible futures after a pandemic, the social transformations that this CoV crisis will bring people, the social changes that CoV will bring people, *online vs.* classroom education, there being no place like school to learn, who being afraid of the ferocious hoax, HCQ or chloroquine (CQ) with or without a macrolide for treatment of COVID-19, a multinational registry analysis, modelling the impact of *social distancing*, testing, contact tracing, household quarantine on second-wave scenarios of COVID-19 epidemic, pandemics meet democracy, experimental evidence from COVID-19 crisis in Spain, the behavioural immune system being designed to avoid infected individuals, not outgroups, targets of T cell responses to SARS-CoV-2 coronavirus in humans with COVID-19 disease, unexposed individuals, SARS-CoV-2 infection protecting *vs.* rechallenge in rhesus macaques, nurses knowing what went wrong in the healthcare (HC) system, the cryo-electron microscopy (EM) structure of SARS-CoV-2 spike in the prefusion conformation, structure, function, antigenicity of SARS-CoV-2 spike glycoprotein, COVID-19 survey, how COVID-19 has affected one's academic life, the effect of large-scale anti-contagion policies on COVID-19 pandemic, whether COVID-19 is increasingly benign, advantages, disadvantages of working on-line for others, the cruel, intense pedagogy of the virus, the first lessons, the analysis of hospital traffic and search engine data in Wuhan, China, indicating early disease activity in the Fall of 2019, homeostasis, coronavirus crisis, human history is a succession of pandemics but people do not learn, COVID-19 reminding people that they are not gods, it being good news, bioinformatics joining the fight *vs.* COVID-19, what people know to date about the transmission of SARS-CoV-2, 10 ideas for a successful digital transit of universities, New Zealand without CoV, five steps to avoid taking steps back, the strategic value of information in the control of epidemics in 20th century, why women resist COVID-19 better, the answer lying on X chromosome, collaboration across disciplines making it easier to solve problems, e.g., COVID-19, learning to care (of each other) in the new time, three topics on technology that should be reviewed, CoV returned women to the domestic sphere, impact on research activity, people must use CoV terrible crisis as an opportunity to rethink the economic system, why children avoid the worst CoV complications might lie in their arteries, the prevalence of asymptomatic SARS-CoV-2 infection, a narrative review, keeping governments accountable, COVID-19 Assessment Scorecard (COVID-SCORE), lessons from the pandemic for EU, the risks of a half-baked integration, ideas for the post-pandemic, the future that awaits people, whether density aggravates COVID-19 Pandemic, early findings, lessons for planners, seroprevalence of immunoglobulin M and G antibodies *vs.* SARS-CoV-2 in China, FDA-approved drug ivermectin inhibiting SARS-CoV-2 replication *in vitro*, the university to come from *remote emergency teaching* to *adapted face-to-face*, that the disease does not overcome life, five lessons from history *vs.* COVID-19, CoV behaving like a sexually transmitted disease (STD), modelling infectious epidemics, CoV jolting laboratories to warp speed, the mind matters, COVID-19, improvise, adapt, overcome, ruxolitinib for the treatment of SARS-CoV-2-induced ARDS and robust T cell immunity in convalescent individuals with asymptomatic or mild COVID-19. González-Candelas group informed the origin of modern syphilis and the emergence of a pandemic *Treponema pallidum* cluster [1]. They reported the molecular epidemiology of human immunodeficiency virus type 1 in the Valencian Community (Spain) and the analysis of transmission clusters [2]. They published the effect of RNA substitution models on viroid and RNA virus phylogenies [3].

On Dec. 31, 2019, Wuhan Municipal Health and Sanitation Commission (Hubei, China) reported on a group of 27 cases of pneumonia of unknown etiology, with common exposure to a seafood, fish and live animal wholesale market in Wuhan City, including seven serious cases. The symptoms of the first case began on Dec. 8, 2019. On Jan. 7, 2020, Chinese authorities identified as a causative agent of the outbreak a new type of virus of the family *Coronaviridae* (SARS-CoV-2), whose genetic sequence was shared by Chinese authorities on Jan. 12. On Mar. 11, World Health Organisation (WHO) declared the global pandemic. The CoVs are a family of viruses that cause infection in humans and a variety of animals [e.g., birds, mammals (camels, cats, bats)]. It is a zoonotic disease, which means that it can be transmitted from animals to humans. The HCoVs can produce clinical symptoms, ranging from the common cold with a seasonal pattern in winter to more serious ones (e.g., those caused by SARS-, MERS-CoVs). Specifically, SARS-CoV-1 in 2003 caused 8 000 cases in 27 countries and a fatality of 10%, and since then it was not detected in humans. Since 2012, 2 500 cases of MERS-CoV were reported in 27 countries (although most cases were detected in Saudi Arabia), with a case fatality of 34%. Most people are infecting with COVID-19 and experiencing respiratory illness. The best way to prevent and slow down transmission is being informed about CoV. Questions, answers and hypotheses (Q/A/H) were proposed on CoVs:

Q1. Genetics and COVID-19: Can genetics explain the variability of response to coronaviruses?

Q2. What is the main risk factor for cancer patients, people with cardiovascular disease (CVD), diabetes and congenital problems?

A2. It is getting old.

Q3. Coronavirus: laboratory virus?

Q4. COVID-19 in cities: How is the pandemic affecting urban health?

Q5. (Bassett and Fogelman, 2013). Is it necessary to reorganize society to achieve a reduction in vulnerability [4]?

Q6. What dilemmas does the pandemic pose for us?

A6. (Kant/Bentham): deontology *vs.* utilitarianism.

A7. Dignity (health) *vs.* price (economy).

A8. Critical thinking *vs.* delegated intelligence.

Q7. (De Sousa Santos, 2020). What potential knowledge about the truth and quality of the institutions of a given society comes from CoV pandemic?

Q8. (De Sousa Santos, 2020). What is the purpose of the goal of permanent crisis?

Q9. (De Sousa Santos, 2020). Surely ideas for possible alternatives are not lacking, but can they lead to political action to achieve them?

H1. Culture has been a fundamental window to support confinement.

The purpose of the present report is to review the pandemic history, etc.

2. Pandemic History: Could People Predict the Coronavirus Pandemic?

Many scientists were waiting for the arrival of a virus as the cause of COVID-19, what they could not predict was when it would happen. The history of other pandemics is revised, and what lessons people can draw from them and, perhaps, what they could have avoided are discussed.

Learning from the past is key to anticipating a disaster as CoV. Table 1 shows the main epidemics in history.

Table 1. The main epidemics in history

Year	1347-1353	1918-1919	1957-1958	1968	1981-	2002-2003	2003-2006	2009-2010	2012	2014-2016	2019-2020
Epidemic	Bubonic plague	Spanish flu (H_1N_1)	Asian flu (H_2N_2)	Hong Kong flu (H_3N_2)	HIV-AIDS	SARS	Avian flu (H_5N_1)	Swine flu (H_1N_1)	MERS	Ebola	COVID-19

3. Meet the Family

The CoVs are a large family of viruses found throughout the world, which cause 30% of upper respiratory tract infections in adults, e.g., *common cold* [5]. The recent COVID-19 outbreak is the third time in 17 years that CoV surfaced. In 2002, SARS-CoV emerged, causing 774 deaths globally before disappearing two years later. In 2012, MERS-CoV led to 1000 and still affects small numbers of people. Meanwhile SARS-CoV-2 was first detected in China in Dec. 2019 and caused >18 000 deaths. The virus is more contagious than its predecessors with early evidence suggesting it is more contagious than seasonal flu.

4. Re/Emerging: Should We Be Ready for the Reemergence of SARS?

The medical and scientific community showed marvelous efforts in the understanding and control of SARS in a short time, as evident by 4 000 publications available online [6]. Despite the achievements, gaps still exist in terms of the molecular basis of the physical stability and transmissibility of this virus, the molecular and immunological basis of disease pathogenesis in humans, screening tests for early or cryptic SARS cases, foolproof infection (*cf.* Figure 1) control procedures for patient care, effective antivirals or antiviral combinations, the usefulness of immunomodulatory agents for late presenters, an effective vaccine with no immune enhancement, and the immediate animal host that transmitted the virus to caged civets in the market at the beginning of the epidemic. The CoVs undergo genetic recombination, which may lead to genotypes and outbreaks. The presence of a large reservoir of SARS-CoV-like viruses in horseshoe bats, together with the culture of eating exotic mammals in southern China, is a time bomb. The possibility of the reemergence of SARS and other viruses from animals or laboratories, and the need for preparedness should not be ignored.

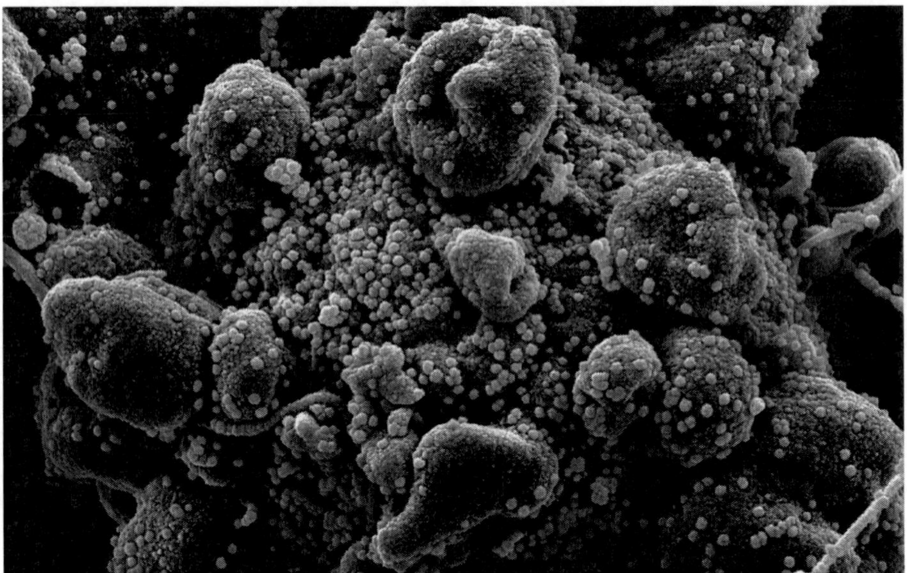

Figure 1. Colourful scanning electron micrograph of an apoptotic cell (*dark green, greyscale*), heavily infected with SARS-CoV-2 particles (*red*), isolated from a sample of a patient. Image captured and enhanced in colour at NIAID Integrated Research Facility (IRF) in Fort Detrick, Maryland.
Source: National Institute of Allergy and Infectious Diseases, JIH.

5. Global Shifts in Mammalian Populations Reveal Key Risk Predictors

Emerging infectious diseases in humans are frequently caused by pathogens originating from animal hosts, and zoonotic disease outbreaks present a major challenge to global health. In order to investigate virus-spillover drivers, the number of viruses mammalian species shared with humans was evaluated [7]. The number of zoonotic viruses detected in mammalian species scales positively with global species abundance, showing that virus transmission risk was the highest from animal species that rose in abundance and expanded their range adapting to human-dominated landscapes. Domesticated species, primates and bats were identified as having more zoonotic viruses than other species. Among threatened wildlife species, those with population reductions because of exploitation and habitat loss shared more viruses with humans. Wildlife exploitation *via* hunting and trade facilitates close wildlife–humans contact, and the findings provide evidence that exploitation, and anthropogenic activities that caused losses in wildlife habitat quality, increased opportunities for animal–human interactions and facilitated zoonotic disease transmission. The study evidences assessing spillover risk from mammalian species and highlights convergent processes whereby the causes of wildlife population declines facilitated animal-virus transmission to humans.

6. The Proximal Origin of SARS-CoV-2

Additional scientific data could swing the balance of evidence to favour one hypothesis over another [8].

Obtaining related viral sequences from animal sources would be the most definitive way of revealing viral origins; e.g., a future observation of an intermediate or fully formed polybasic cleavage site in a SARS-CoV-2-like virus from animals would lend even support to the natural-selection (NS) hypotheses. It would also be helpful to obtain more genetic and functional data about SARS-CoV-2, e.g., animal studies. The identification of a potential intermediate host of SARS-CoV-2, and sequencing of the virus from early cases, would similarly be highly informative. Irrespective of the exact mechanisms by which SARS-CoV-2 originated *via* NS, the ongoing surveillance of pneumonia in humans and other animals is clearly of utmost importance. The emergence and rapid global spread of SARS-CoV-2 mark 3rd identification of a CoV capable of causing severe, potentially fatal disease in humans in 21st century [9]. After Andersen et al., the sequencing of proximal zoonotic ancestors to SARS-CoV-2 aided in the identification of alleles that may contribute to the virus' virulence in humans.

7. An Interactive Web-Based Dashboard to Track COVID-19 in Real Time

In response to SARS-CoV-2 ongoing PH emergency, an online interactive dashboard, hosted by the Center for Systems Science and Engineering (CSSE) at Johns Hopkins University, Baltimore, MD, US, was developed to visualise and track reported cases of COVID-19 in RT [10]. The dashboard, first shared publicly on Jan. 22, 2020, illustrates the location and number of confirmed COVID-19 cases, deaths and recoveries for all affected countries. It was developed to provide researchers, PH authorities and the general public with a user-friendly tool to track the outbreak as it unfolds. All data collected and displayed are made freely available, *via* Google Sheets and a GitHub repository, and the feature layers of the dashboard, which are included in Esri Living Atlas.

8. Scientific Analysis of Past, Current and Future Situation of Pandemic

The world is experiencing a major pandemic caused by SARS-CoV-2, CoV causing COVID-19 [11]. The disease first entered the human population in Hubei province, China, in mid-November 2019 and manifested in Wuhan, the largest metropolitan area of Hubei, when a cluster of patients were admitted to hospital with a *severe pneumonia of unknown cause* in early December. Although humanity survived previous pandemics by infectious agents, the present one is unprecedented in its capacity to take advantage of modern globalization, allowing for massive transborder spread at a surprising speed. The pandemic affects 217 countries and territories, with 12 000 000 infected subjects, 500 000 deaths and 6 000 000 recovered patients.

9. Analysis of the Most Promising SARS-CoV-2 Drug Available to Date

A coalition of PH experts, doctors and scientists worldwide drew attention to the need for high-quality evaluation protocols of the potential beneficial effect of HCQ (*cf.* Figure 2), as a post-exposure drug for exposed people, i.e., people with close contact with positive tested (*cf.* Figure 3) patients (e.g., home, medical caregivers) [12].

They reviewed HCQ mechanisms of antiviral effect, risk-benefit ratio taking into consideration pharmacokinetics/pharmacodynamics and efficacy thresholds. They studied its use as an antimalarial, an antiviral and an immunomodulating drug, and concluded that the use of HCQ at doses matching that of the standard treatment of systemic lupus erythematous, which proved safety and efficacy in terms of HCQ blood and tissue concentration adapted to bodyweight, at $6 mg \cdot kg^{-1} \cdot d^{-1}$ one (loading dose) followed by $5 mg \cdot kg^{-1} \cdot d^{-1}$, with a maximum limit of $600 mg \cdot d^{-1}$ in all cases should swiftly be clinically evaluated as a post-exposure drug for exposed people.

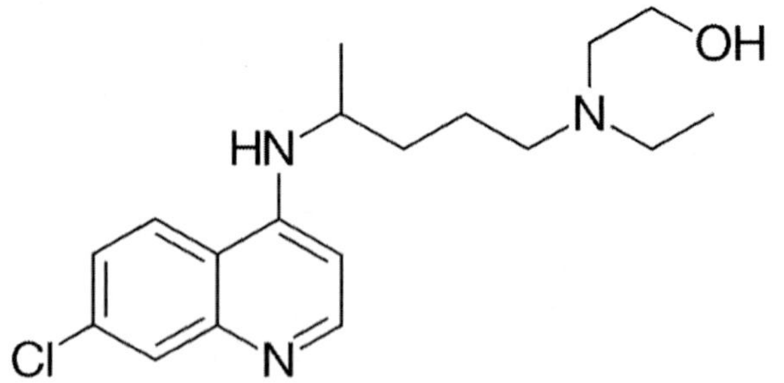

Figure 2. Molecular structure of hydroxychloroquine.

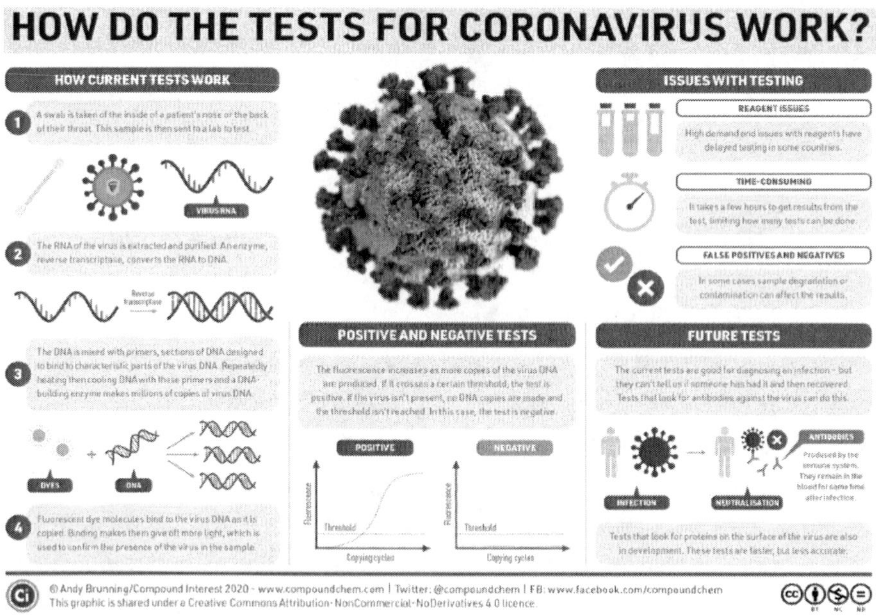

Figure 3. How do the tests for coronavirus work?
Source: Andy Brunning/Compound Interest 2020.

10. Drug Repurposing for CoV Treatment: A Molecular Topology Study

A communication illustrated the results of a computational study based on MT, focused on the drugs repositioning to treat SARS-CoV-2, responsible for COVID-19 [13]. *Via* lopinavir, a well-known viral protease (*cf.* Figure 4) inhibitor as the reference drug, a mathematical pattern was found allowing the screening of the marketed drugs, searching for potential candidates to inhibit said enzyme (*cf.* Figure 5).

This way, possible therapeutic alternatives to fight CoV are found. Results indicate that antivirals, e.g., brecanavir, and a number of groups of drugs, among which antibiotics of the macrolide family (azithromycin, clarithromycin, erythromycin, etc.) stand, could be useful in treating COVID-19 infection.

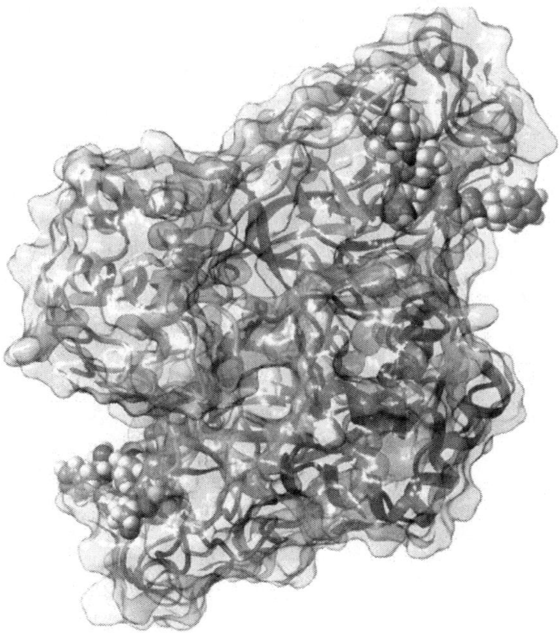

Figure 4. Main protease (Mpro) of the SARS-CoV-2 virus.

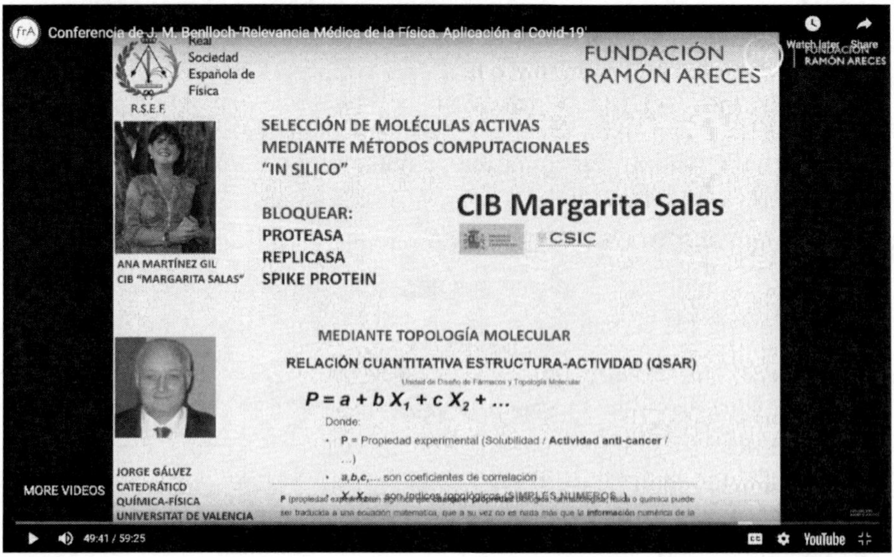

Figure 5. Molecular topology: Quantitative structure-activity relationship. Source: J.M. Benlloch.

11. Mathematics to Explain the Measures against the Coronavirus

Starting from a low number of those infected with the new CoV, in a short time a large number of infected people who cannot assimilate the health system may exist, which is reflected in the mathematical curves of exponential growth, a reality that the population accepts and forced the Spanish Government to adopt extraordinary measures to contain the pandemic [14].

12. The Curve: Why Is the COVID-19 Curve so Important?

Exasperated many people are by governments' response to COVID-19, such decisions are ultimately political. People must hold politicians to account for PH shortcomings, and recognise and value the complex specialist work that disease modellers undertake. *The Rules of Contagion* is a timely reminder of the importance of disease modelling [15]. Without such models, people would be in far greater trouble battling COVID-19 [16]. The epidemic presents many variables. However, four letters are key (DOTS):

D, duration;
O, opportunity:
T, transmissibility;
S, susceptibility.

By lowering the opportunity, people will be able to stop the COVID-19 curve.

13. Can a Virus Undermine Human Rights?

How can humans think about health crisis management systems that protect society without undermining individual freedom (*cf.* Figure 6) [17]? National legislatures should adopt adequate rules to ensure that health surveillance and monitoring policies will be strictly prescribed by law, proportionate to PH necessities, done in a transparent manner, controlled by independent regulation authorities, subject to constant ethical reflection, non-discriminatory and respectful of fundamental HRs.

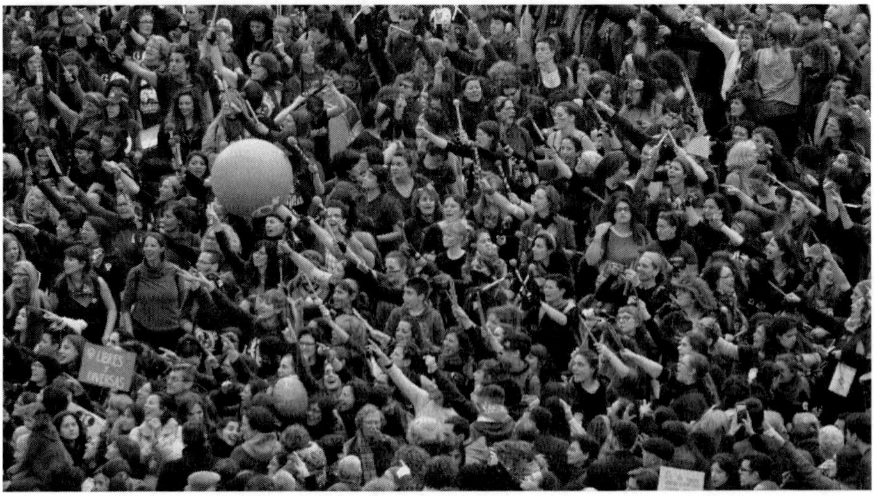

Figure 6. Demonstration in times of epidemic.
Source: Radiotelevisión Española (RTVE).

14. Answering the Right Questions for Policymakers on COVID-19

The key questions that officials and experts in US need to be able to address were identified [18]: 1) clinical presentation and testing; 2) treatment: supplies, hospital beds, workforce; 3) non-pharmaceutical interventions: adherence and mobility (*cf.* Figure 7); 4) PH response: ability to contact trace and identify exposures; 5) compound hazards and concurrent hazard planning. Questions require dedicated modelling work, but all are basic data questions. Although the questions are focused on the current needs in US, informed by what people were asked by the state and local response, the same core challenges are being faced everywhere that the outbreak hits. As a community of practice, people will have to continue to keep up with frontline decision-making needs. Someone will have to load ventilators into a plane, which are the numbers that will save lives.

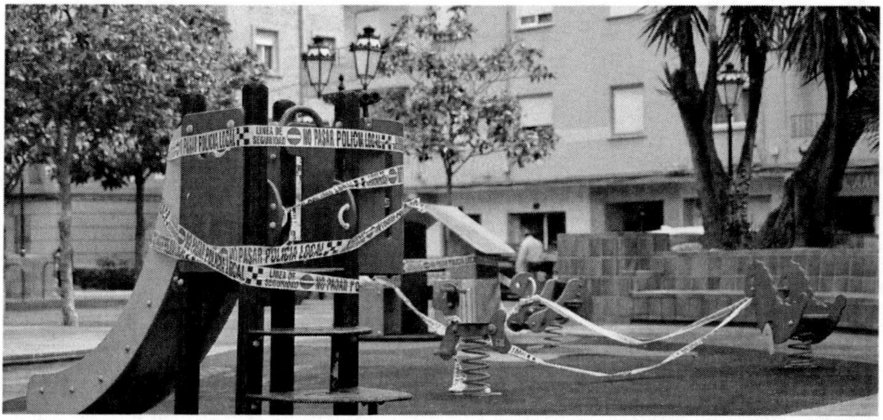

Figure 7. Confinement of Spanish children imposed by COVID-19.
Source: RTVE.

15. Building Trust Influencing Online COVID-19 Content in Social Media

Because many are turning to social media for information and advice, the differentiation between individuals who are qualified to provide accurate information online and *armchair epidemiologists* results risingly difficult [19]. Members of the lay public might try to identify the most seemingly qualified member of their close net as a trusted resource to vet information, which individuals might feel unequipped to respond effectively to misinformation that individuals are exposed to on social media (*cf.* Figure 8). To dispel myths, one strategy for the lay public and trusted sources of information, i.e., epidemiologists, is inoculation, which, in this sense, focuses on strengthening a person's attitudes and opinions to protect them from misinformation; e.g., a common myth circulating on social media is that COVID-19 was engineered in a laboratory. Affirming the proliferation of misinformation about COVID-19, one can point to the use of conspiracy theory rhetoric, which characteristically shows unsubstantiated links and invokes themes of unseen nefarious nets that act behind the scenes of the pandemic. Owing to the ubiquitous nature of

COVID-19 misinformation, all members of the broad digital social nets (e.g., government agencies, social media companies, HC providers, consumers or propagators of information themselves) share in the responsibility to help address the broader implications of the pandemic and the underlying infodemic to strengthen community resiliency.

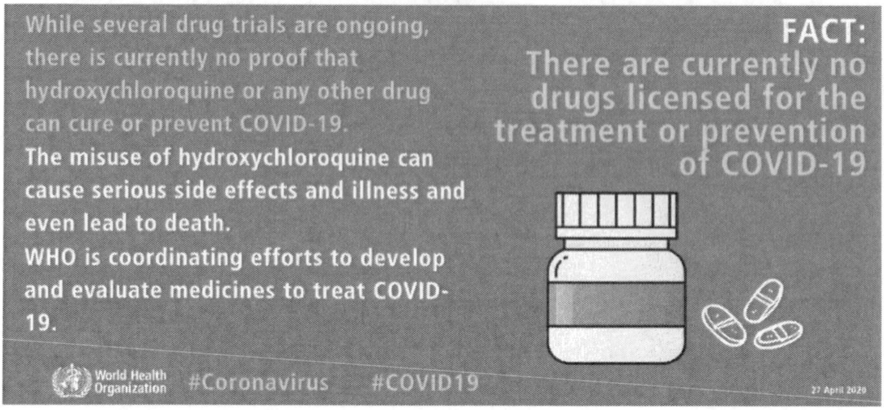

Figure 8. There are currently no drugs licensed for COVID-19 treatment or prevention. Source: WHO.

16. Ethnicity and COVID-19: An Urgent Public Health Research Priority

Black and minority ethnic communities might be at risen risk of acquisition, disease severity and poor outcomes in COVID-19. Specific ethnic groups, *e,g*., south Asians, present higher rates of some comorbidities (*e,g*., diabetes, hypertension, CVDs), which were associated with severe disease and mortality in COVID-19. Ethnicity could interplay with virus spread *via* cultural, behavioural and societal differences (e.g., lower socioeconomic status, health-seeking behaviour, intergenerational cohabitation). Disentangling the relative importance of the factors requires prospective studies, focusing on quantifying absolute risks and outcomes, and qualitative studies of behaviours and responses to pandemic control messages. If ethnicity is found to be associated with adverse COVID-19 outcomes, this must directly, and urgently, inform PH interventions globally [20].

17. Now/Forecasting Potential Domestic/International SARS-CoV-2 Spread

Since Dec. 31, 2019, Chinese city of Wuhan reported an outbreak of atypical pneumonia caused by SARS-CoV-2. Cases were exported to other Chinese cities and internationally, threatening to trigger a global outbreak. An estimate of the size of the epidemic in Wuhan was provided based on the number of cases exported from Wuhan to cities outside mainland China, and the extent of the domestic and global PH risks of epidemics was forecasted, accounting for social and non-pharmaceutical prevention interventions [21]. Data Dec. 31, 2019–Jan. 28, 2020 on the number of cases exported from Wuhan internationally (known days of symptom onset Dec. 25, 2019–Jan. 19, 2020) were used to infer the number of infections in Wuhan Dec. 1, 2019–Jan. 25, 2020. Cases exported domestically were estimated. The national and global spread of SARS-CoV-2 was forecasted, accounting for the effect of the metropolitan-wide quarantine of Wuhan and surrounding cities, which began Jan. 23–24, 2020. Data on monthly flight bookings from Official Aviation Guide and human mobility across more than 300 prefecture-level cities in mainland China from the Tencent database were used. Data on confirmed cases were obtained from the reports published by the Chinese Center for Disease Control and Prevention. Serial interval estimates were based on previous studies of SARS-CoV. A susceptible-exposed-infectious-recovered metapopulation model was used to simulate the epidemics across all major cities in China. The basic reproductive number was estimated *via* Markov Chain Monte Carlo methods and presented *via* the resulting posterior mean and 95% credible interval. In the baseline scenario, it was estimated that the basic reproductive number for SARS-CoV-2 was 2.68 and 75 815 individuals were infected in Wuhan as of Jan. 25, 2020. The epidemic doubling time was 6.4d. In the baseline scenario, Chongqing, Beijing, Shanghai, Guangzhou and Shenzhen were estimated to import 461, 113, 98, 111 and 80 infections from Wuhan, respectively. If the transmissibility of SARS-CoV-2 were similar everywhere domestically and over time, epidemics were inferred to be growing exponentially in multiple major cities of China with a lag time behind the Wuhan outbreak of about 1–2 weeks. Given that SARS-CoV-2 is no longer contained in Wuhan, other major Chinese cities are probably sustaining localised outbreaks. Large cities overseas with close transport links to China could become outbreak epicentres, unless substantial PH interventions at the population and personal levels be implemented immediately. Independent self-sustaining outbreaks in major cities globally could become inevitable, because of substantial exportation of presymptomatic cases and in the absence of large-scale PH interventions. Preparedness plans and mitigation interventions should be readied for quick deployment globally.

18. Offline: COVID-19 and the NHS—A National Scandal

National health Service (NHS) was wholly unprepared for the pandemic [22]. It is impossible to understand why. Based on their modelling of the Wuhan outbreak of COVID-19, Wu et al. wrote in *The Lancet* on Jan. 31, 2020:

> On the present trajectory, 2019-nCoV could be about to become a global epidemic... for health protection within China and internationally... preparedness plans should be readied for deployment at short notice, including securing supply chains of pharmaceuticals, personal protective equipment (PPE), hospital supplies, and the necessary human resources to deal with the consequences of a global outbreak of this magnitude.

The warning was not made lightly. It should have been read by the Chief Medical Officer, Chief Executive Officer of NHS in England and

Chief Scientific Adviser. They had a duty to immediately put NHS and British public on high alert. February should have been used to expand CoV testing capacity, ensure the distribution of WHO-approved PPE, and establish training programmes and guidelines to protect NHS staff. They did not take any action. The result was chaos and panic across NHS. Patients will die unnecessarily. Staff of NHS will die unnecessarily. It is, indeed, as one health worker wrote, *a national scandal*. The gravity of that scandal must be understood.

19. The Novel CoV Outbreak: What People Know and What They Do Not

The lack of diagnostics that could be rapidly adapted for SARS-CoV-2 puts already vulnerable countries at an even higher risk, and strains weak health systems during epi- and pandemics. Investment in smart diagnostics that could be rapidly applied to emerging pathogens on a large scale is needed and needs to be prioritized by stakeholders [23].

20. COVID-19: Navigating Uncertainties Together

As proponents of science, people can make the best of the grave situation (*cf.* Figure 9) [24]. People may not be able to stop dangerous pathogens from emerging, but they can certainly be better informed and more prepared. As society is forced to confront the importance of the science scientists do and love, people should be advocating for more and consistent science funding, and stronger science voices in government. People should publicly support and encourage the people putting in tireless effort to study the virus, fight misinformation, care for the sick, and work to treatments and vaccines. They should take advantage of disrupted routines to pause, spend time with loved ones, think and re-think. Plenty of research shows that pressure drives auspicious evolution, and time to step back and contemplate is essential for creativity and innovation. People may consider using downtime they might have to evaluate research directions, write up results, or realize ideas they may have tabled for literature reviews or other thought pieces.

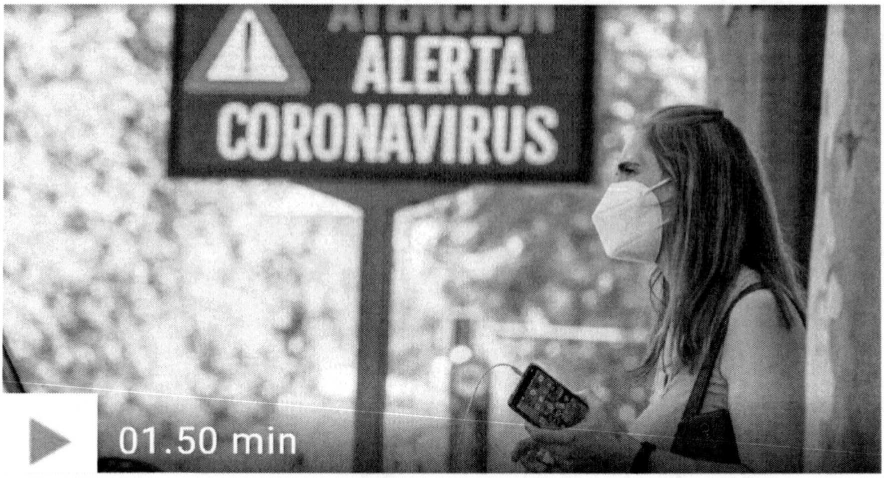

Figure 9. Attention: Coronavirus Alert. Source: RTVE.

21. COVID-19 Is a Data Science Issue

People must remember that behind the numbers are human lives. Real people who are worried and afraid for themselves or for their loved ones. It is easy enough to calculate a mortality curve that show that it is those who are ≥60 years old, or suffer from pre-existing conditions, are the most likely to die. It is another thing to realize that the figures show that it is your aged parents or grandparents, or immunocompromised friends and family, who are most at risk. People live in challenging times, but with the right data, and the right science, they can make a difference [25].

22. Differentiating COVID-19 Response Strategies

Pandemic of COVID-19 is the first in 21st century, which has and will continue to bring many changes to the global. While the implementation of basic strategies (e.g., population sensitization about preventive measures) must be global, countries in different regions must consider their specific situations and develop effective tailored prevention strategies, based on the price China paid and learned lessons [26].

23. COVID-19

The COVID-19 is a novel respiratory illness caused by SARS-CoV-2 [27]. Viral entry is mediated *via* viral spike protein and host ACE2 enzyme interaction. Most cases are mild; severe disease usually involves cytokine storm and organ failure. Therapeutics (e.g., antivirals, immunomodulators, vaccines) are in development.

24. Imbalanced Host Response to SARS-CoV-2 Drives Development of COVID-19

Viral pandemics, e.g., that caused by SARS-CoV-2, pose an imminent threat to humanity. Owing to its recent emergence, a paucity of information regarding viral behaviour and host response following SARS-CoV-2 infection exists. An in-depth analysis of the transcriptional response to SARS-CoV-2 as it compares to other respiratory viruses is offered [28]. Cell and animal models of SARS-CoV-2 infections, and transcriptional and serum profiling of COVID-19 patients, consistently revealed a unique and inappropriate inflammatory response, which is defined by low levels of type-I and -III interferons juxtaposed to elevated chemokines and high expression of interleukin 6 (IL-6). Reduced innate antiviral defenses coupled with exuberant inflammatory cytokine production are the defining and driving COVID-19 feature.

25. A Multibasic Cleavage Site in the Spike Protein of SARS-CoV-2 Is Essential

The pandemic SARS-CoV-2 threatens PH worldwide. The viral spike protein mediates SARS-CoV-2 entry into host cells and harbours an S1/S2 cleavage site containing multiple arginine residues (multibasic) not found in closely related animal CoVs. However, the role of the multibasic cleavage site in SARS-CoV-2 infection is unknown. The cellular protease furin cleaves the spike protein at S1/S2 site and cleavage is essential for S protein-mediated cell-cell fusion and entry into human lung cells [29]. Moreover, optimizing S1/S2 site increased cell-cell but not virus-cell fusion, showing that the corresponding viral variants might exhibit increased cell-cell spread and potentially altered virulence. Acquisition of an S1/S2 multibasic cleavage site was essential for SARS-CoV-2 infection of humans and furin was identified as a potential target for therapeutic intervention.

26. SARS-CoV-2 Receptor ACE2 Is an Interferon-Stimulated Gene

Pressing urgency exists to understand the pathogenesis of SARS-CoV-2, which causes COVID-19. Spike (S) protein of SARS-CoV-2 binds ACE2 and, in concert with host proteases, principally TMPRSS2, promotes cellular entry. The cell subsets targeted by SARS-CoV-2 in host tissues, and the factors that regulate *ACE2* expression, remain unknown. Human, non-human primate and mouse single-cell RNA-sequencing (scRNA-seq) datasets were leveraged across health and disease to uncover putative SARS-CoV-2 targets amongst tissue-resident cell subsets [30]. The *ACE2* and *TMPRSS2* co-expressing cells were identified in lung type-II pneumocytes, ileal absorptive enterocytes and nasal goblet secretory cells. Strikingly, *ACE2* is a human interferon-stimulated gene *in vitro via* airway epithelial cells, and the findings were extended to *in vivo* viral infections. The SARS-CoV-2 exploits species-specific interferon-driven upregulation of *ACE2*, a tissue-protective mediator during lung injury, to enhance infection.

27. SARS-CoV-2 Evolutionary Analysis Rejects Recent Recombination Event

Novel SARS-CoV-2 associated with human to human transmission and severe human infection was recently reported from Wuhan City, China [31]. The objectives were to characterize the genetic relations of SARS-CoV-2 and to search for putative recombination within the subgenus of sarbecovirus. Putative recombination was investigated by RDP4 and Simplot vs. 3.5.1, and discordant phylogenetic clustering in individual genomic fragments was confirmed by phylogenetic analysis *via* maximum likelihood and Bayesian methods. The SARS-CoV-2, although closely related to BatCoV RaTG13 sequence throughout the genome, shows discordant clustering with Bat_SARS-like CoV sequences. Specifically, in the 5′-part spanning the first 11 498 nucleotides and the last 3′-part spanning 24 341–30 696 positions, SARS-CoV-2 and RaTG13 formed a single cluster with Bat_SARS-like CoV sequences, whereas in the middle region spanning the 3′-end of open reading frame (ORF)1a, ORF1b and almost half of the spike regions, SARS-CoV-2 and RaTG13 grouped in a separate distant lineage in the sarbecovirus branch. The levels of genetic similarity between SARS-CoV-2 and RaTG13 show that the latter does not provide the exact variant that caused humans outbreak, but the hypothesis that SARS-CoV-2 originated from bats is likely. The novel SARS-CoV-2 is not-mosaic consisting in half of its genome of a distinct lineage in β-

CoV. The genomic features, and their potential association with virus characteristics and virulence in humans need attention.

28. SARS-CoV-2 Pathogenicity and Transmissibility: Comparison with Viruses

Zoonotic SARS-CoV-2 was identified as the causative agent of the viral pneumonia outbreak in Wuhan, China, at the end of 2019. Although SARS-CoV-2 can cause a severe respiratory illness (e.g., SARS, MERS), evidence from clinics showed that it is generally less pathogenic than SARS-CoV and much less than MERS-CoV. Transmissibility of SARS-CoV-2 is still debated and needs to be assessed. In order to avoid SARS-CoV-2 outbreak turning into an epidemic or pandemic, and minimize the mortality rate, China activated emergency response procedures, but much remains to be learned about the features of the virus to refine the risk assessment and response. The current knowledge in SARS-CoV-2 pathogenicity and transmissibility was summarized in comparison with several commonly known emerging viruses, and information urgently needed for a better control of the disease was highlighted [32].

29. SARS-Coronavirus 2 and COVID 2019: The Epidemic and the Challenges

Emergence of COVID-19 in China at the end of 2019 caused a large global outbreak and is a major PH issue [33]. As of Feb. 11, 2020, data from WHO showed that more than 43 000 confirmed cases were identified in 28 countries/regions, with >99% of cases being detected in China. On Jan. 30, 2020, WHO declared COVID-19 as 6th PH emergency of international concern. The SARS-CoV-2 is closely related to two bat-derived severe acute respiratory syndrome-like CoVs, bat-SL-CoVZC45 and bat-SL-CoVZXC21. It is spread by human-to-human transmission *via* droplets or direct contact, and infection was estimated to present mean incubation period of 6.4 days and a basic reproduction number R_0 of 2.24–3.58. Among patients with pneumonia caused by SARS-CoV-2, fever was the most common symptom, followed by cough. Bilateral lung involvement with ground-glass opacity was the most common finding from computed tomography images of the chest. The case of SARS-CoV-2 pneumonia in US is responding well to remdesivir, which is undergoing a CT in China. Controlling infection to prevent SARS-CoV-2 spread is the primary intervention. However, PH authorities must keep monitoring the situation closely, as the more people can learn about the novel virus and its associated outbreak, the better they can respond.

30. Insights into 2019 Novel Coronavirus in Light of Past Human Outbreaks

The CoVs are RNA viruses that became a major PH concern since SARS-CoV outbreak in 2002. The continuous CoVs evolution was highlighted with the emergence of MERS-CoV outbreak in 2012. The world is concerned about SARS-CoV-2 that was initially identified in Wuhan City, China in Dec. 2019. Patients presented with severe viral pneumonia and respiratory illness. The number of cases was mounting since then. As of late Feb. 2020, tens of thousands of cases and several thousand deaths were reported in China, and thousands of cases in other countries. Although SARS-CoV-2 fatality rate is lower than SARS-CoV, the virus seems to be highly contagious based on the number of infected cases to date. Structure, genome organization and CoVs entry into target cells were discussed, and insights into past and present outbreaks were provided [34]. The future of HCoV outbreaks will not only depend on how the viruses will evolve, but also on how people develop efficient prevention and treatment strategies to deal with the continuous threat.

31. Insight into 2019 Coronavirus: Lessons from SARS-CoV and MERS-COV

The rapid COVID-19 spread, caused by a zoonotic β-CoV (SARS-CoV-2), became a global threat. Awareness of SARS-CoV-2 biofeatures should be updated in time and needs to be comprehensively summarized to help optimise control measures and make therapeutic decisions. Based on recently published literature, official documents and selected up-to-date preprint studies, SARS-CoV-2-infection virology, and origin, epidemiology, clinical manifestations, pathology and treatment were reviewed in comparison with SARS- and MERS-CoV infection [35]. Genome of SARS-CoV-2 partially resembled SARS/MERS-CoV and indicated a bat origin. The COVID-19 generally presented a high reproductive number, a long incubation period, a short serial interval and a low case fatality rate (much higher in patients with comorbidities) than SARS/MERS. Clinical presentation and pathology of COVID-19 greatly resembled SARS/MERS, with less upper respiratory and gastrointestinal symptoms, and more exudative lesions in post-mortems. Potential treatments included remdesivir, CQ, tocilizumab, convalescent plasma and vaccine immunization. The initial experience from the current pandemic and lessons from the previous two pandemics can help improve future preparedness plans and combat disease progression.

32. COVID-19 Sex-Bias: A Meta-Analysis and Review in Disease and Immunity

Anecdotal reports of a male sex bias in COVID-19 existed. A meta-analysis of available case reports was performed to investigate if a difference existed in the proportion of males and females infected with COVID-19 and sex associated with a difference in risk of intensive treatment unit (ITU) admission or death [36]. A meta-analysis of 29 reports was performed. An internet search was performed for reports in any language that included sex as a variable when describing case numbers, ITU admissions or death between Jan. 1–Mar. 30, 2020. Reports were excluded if they did not report the sex difference in overall case numbers or where possible duplication existed. Summary level data were extracted from reports. Meta-analyses were assessed the proportion of males and females in total numbers of confirmed cases, estimate odds ratios with 95% confidence interval associated with sex for ITU admission and death, based on pooled average effect measures that were weighted according to the size and precision of each report. Fixed and random effects models were estimated. A total of 29 studies were eligible with a total of 206 128 cases. The proportion of male cases with COVID-19 was 0.52. Male sex associated with an increased risk of ITU admission. Male sex associated with an increased risk of mortality.

33. COVID-19 Evolves in Human Hosts

People are threatened by an unprecedented pandemic: COVID-19. How different is it from other CoVs? Will it be attenuated or become more virulent? Which animals may be its original host? A total of 377 publicly available complete genome sequences for COVID-19 virus, previously known flu-causing CoVs (HCov-229E, HCov-OC43, HCov-NL63, HCov-HKU1), and lethal, pathogenic viruses, SARS, MERS, Victoria, Lassa, Yamagata, Ebola and Dengue were analised [37]. Strong similarities between the current circulating COVID-19, and SARS and MERS, and COVID-19 in rhinolophines and pangolins were found. On the contrary, COVID-19 shares little similarity with the flu-causing CoVs and the other known viruses. Strikingly, divergence of COVID-19 strains isolated from human hosts steadily rose Dec. 2019–Mar. 2020, showing COVID-19 is actively evolving in human hosts. From all existing human COVID-19 genome sequences, the first common model that represents the shared sequences of the human COVID-19 strains was calculated, which provides important information for vaccine and Ab development. Geographic and time-course analysis of the evolutionary trees of the human COVID-19 reveals possible evolutional paths among strains from 21 countries, which finding presents important implications to COVID-19 management and vaccines development.

34. COVID-19: A Lesson in Humility and Opportunity for Sagacity and Hope

People must never forget the importance of being humble and sagacious, individually and as a society [38]. They are witnessing glimmers of hope. People are proud to see the courage they witnessed by researchers and clinical care teams, showing a fortitude that they are sure will lead to a better future.

35. COVID-19: The Isolation That Has Brought People Together

It is soon for people to know where this *war* will take them, or its full impact on their professional lives, patients and families [39]. However, the one thing people discovered is that isolation will not separate them. Stronger together, people press on.

36. A Real-Time Dashboard of Clinical Trials for COVID-19

Over 500 CTs were registered at the various international and national CT registry sites. Findings from randomised CTs that were published investigated the efficacy of lopinavir–ritonavir compared to standard of care, HCQ to best supportive care, favipiravir to arbidol and lopinavir–ritonavir to arbidol. Other non-randomised CTs investigated HCQ *vs.* HCQ combined with azithromycin. Over 300 CTs enrol participants, and cover further investigations of the drugs and promising therapies [e.g., remdesivir, IL-6 inhibitors (tocilizumab, sarilumab), convalescent plasma therapy, stem-cell transfusion, vaccine candidates, several other well-known direct acting antivirals, traditional Chinese medicines]. Most CTs will offer comparative efficacy data *vs.* standard of care according to local COVID-19 treatment guidelines, but a handful of randomized controlled CTs will provide head-to-head evidence between high profile interventions. The net of completed, ongoing and planned COVID-19 interventional CTs of the interventions or intervention groups that are explored in two CTs was informed [40].

37. COVID-19: New Virus, but Familiar Receptor/Cytokine Release Syndrome

Zhou et al. [41] and Hoffmann et al. [42] identified ACE2 as an SARS-CoV-2 receptor, and the latter showed its entry mechanism depends on cellular transmembrane serine protease 2 (TMPRSS2), which results may explain proinflammatory cytokine release *via* the associated angiotestin II pathway and a possible therapeutic target *via* the IL-6-STAT3 axis [43].

38. Impact of Contact Tracing on SARS-CoV-2 Transmission

As people look to post-lockdown strategies, they must examine the experience of countries that successfully controlled SARS-CoV2 transmission or present low mortality (e.g., China, Singapore, Taiwan, SK, Germany, Iceland, *cf.* Figure 10) [44]. Successful strategies include ample testing and contact tracing, supplemented by moderate forms of *social distancing*. Contact tracing on the scale that is needed for SARS-CoV-2 response is labour intensive, and imperfect if done manually. Technology-based approaches result greatly needed to assist in identification of contacts, especially if case detection is aggressive. Building on SARS-CoV-2 experience in Shenzhen and other settings, enhanced case finding and contact tracing must be part of the long-term response to the pandemic, which can get people most of the way to control.

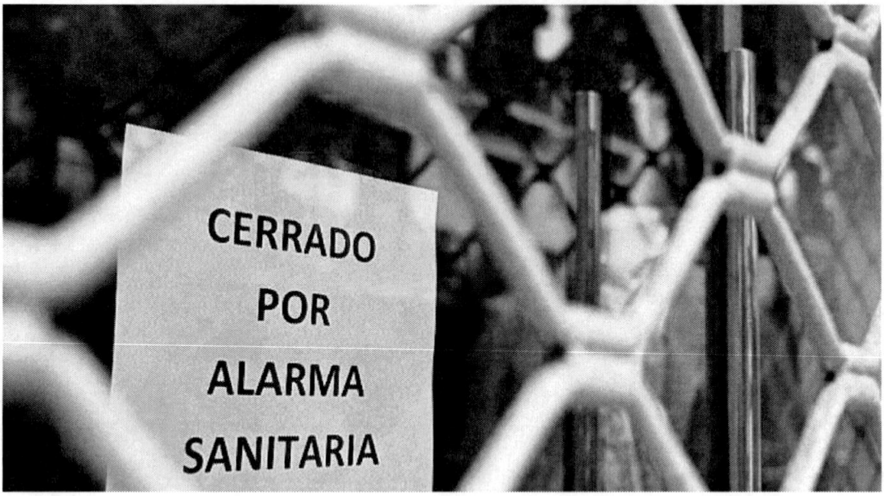

Figure 10. CLOSED FOR HEALTH ALARM. Source: RTVE.

39. What Policy Makers Need to Know About COVID-19 Protective Immunity

Researchers must be commended for decades of iterative efforts, bringing people to a point where many candidate vaccines exist in development *vs.* a virus first sequenced in Jan., 2020 [45]. Delivery of efficacious vaccines is not a competitive race to the finish, but a considered evaluation of a safe, potent, global response. Few would disagree that science must guide the clinical therapeutic approach to an infected person. Science must also guide policy decisions. Reliance on comprehensive seroprevalence data and a solid, research-based grasp of correlates of protection will allow policy to be guided by secure, evidence-based assumptions on herd immunity, rather than optimistic guesses.

40. Isolation and Inclusion

In times of crisis, research might seem a low priority, but as with all crises, it is essential that people monitor innovations and collect high-quality data so that, at a later date, they can learn what worked and what did not (*cf.* Figure 11) [46]. Such research must be done, as far as possible, according to normal standards and complying with ethical best practice. It is important that the invaluable resources of longitudinal cohort studies around the world be maintained as much as possible, because they will be essential when people have time to examine the long-term consequences of COVID-19 pandemic for their mental health. People's world of social isolation was never so inclusive: once the pandemic passed, may the benefits endure and the disadvantages fade away.

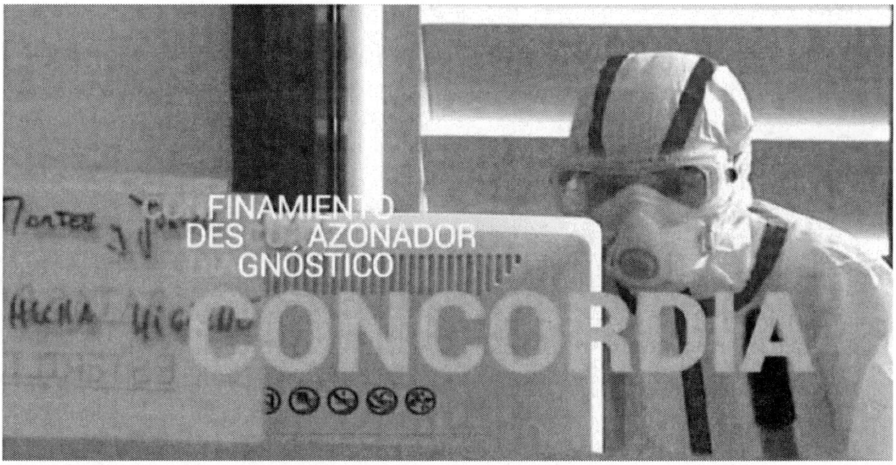

Figure 11. The Cervantes Institute proposes to transform words that overwhelm us. Source: RTVE.

41. Key Ethical Questions for Reseach during the COVID-19 Pandemic

For all research to be considered ethical, the benefits must be high and the risk minimized [47]. The research community must be clear about who will benefit from the research, how it can be implemented to inform policy and practice, and in what time frame. Ethics committees across the globe present a vital role to play in weighing the issues and context of a growing plethora of online studies. Given *social distancing* and lockdowns, an effective digital response is crucial. Clinical mental health services globally must mobilise staff digitally and remotely to meet current need. The research community needs to respond effectively to COVID-19 pandemic, but people must ensure that what they are doing is ethical.

42. Virtual Treatment and Social Distancing

The setting is a painful but powerful moment for psychotherapy [48]. Patients need therapy more than ever, yet are physically distanced from it. Psychotherapy might be harder in respects to do at a distance, but teletherapy does work, and the basic principles remain the same. The interpersonal, environmental context can provide a useful frame for treating the problems patients face.

43. Public Health Messaging and Harm Reduction in the Time of COVID-19

As a society, people can protect vulnerable populations by practising PH and prevention-science fundamentals [49]. People have a moral, societal and professional responsibility to ensure that those living on the margins are not left out of the efforts.

44. Decolonising COVID-19

Territorial colonialism may have ended long ago, but the contemporary global health crisis can serve as a reminder that the colonisation of medicine, economics and politics, remains alive [50]. People must reflect on practices that have their origins in 19th century imperialism and replace them with systems that are rooted in values of recognition, reciprocity and respect.

45. Trained Immunity: Tool Reducing SARS-CoV-2 Susceptibility and Severity

Infection of SARS-CoV-2 is mild in most individuals but progresses into severe pneumonia in a small proportion of patients [51]. The risen susceptibility to severe disease in the elderly and individuals with co-morbidities argues for an initial defect in anti-viral host defense mechanisms. Long-term boosting of innate immune responses (*trained immunity*) by certain live vaccines [bacillus Calmette-Guérin (BCG), oral polio vaccine, measles] induces heterologous protection *vs.* infections, *via* epigenetic, transcriptional and functional reprogramming of innate immune cells. Induction of trained immunity by whole microorganism vaccines may represent an important tool for reducing susceptibility and severity to SARS-CoV-2.

46. Herd Immunity: Understanding COVID-19

In a sufficiently immune population, herd immunity provides indirect protection to susceptible individuals by minimizing the probability of an effective contact between a susceptible individual and an infected host [52]. In its simplest form, herd immunity will begin to take effect when a population reaches the herd immunity threshold, i.e., when the proportion of individuals who result immune to the pathogen crosses $1 - 1/R_0$. At this point, sustained transmission cannot occur, so the outbreak will decline. However, in real-world populations, the situation is usually much more complex. Epidemiological and immunological factors (e.g., population structure, variation in transmission dynamics between populations, waning immunity) will lead to variation in the extent of indirect protection conferred by herd immunity, which aspects must be taken into account when discussing the establishment of herd immunity in populations. Possible approaches exist to build widespread SARS-CoV-2 immunity: 1) a mass vaccination campaign, which requires the development of an effective and safe vaccine, or 2) natural immunization of global populations with the virus over time. However, the consequences of the latter are serious and far-reaching (a large fraction of the human population would need to become infected with the virus and millions would succumb to it). In the absence of a vaccination program, establishing herd immunity should not be the ultimate goal. Instead, an emphasis should be placed on policies that protect the most vulnerable groups, in the hopes that herd immunity will eventually be achieved as a byproduct of such measures, although not the primary objective itself.

47. Clinical Features of Patients Infected with 2019 CoV in Wuhan, China

A recent cluster of pneumonia cases in Wuhan, China, was caused by a novel β-CoV, SARS-CoV-2. The epidemiological, clinical, laboratory, and radiological characteristics, and treatment and clinical outcomes of the patients were reported [53]. All patients with suspected SARS-CoV-2 were admitted to a designated hospital in Wuhan. Data on patients with laboratory-confirmed SARS-CoV-2 infection by RT-polymerase chain reaction (PCR) and next-generation sequencing (NGS) were prospectively collected and analysed. Data were obtained with standardised data collection forms shared by WHO and the International Severe Acute

Respiratory and Emerging Infection Consortium from electronic medical records. Researchers directly communicated with patients or their families to ascertain epidemiological and symptom data. Outcomes were compared between patients who were admitted to ICU and those who had not. Infection of SARS-CoV-2 caused clusters of severe respiratory illness similar to SARS-CoV and was associated with ICU admission and high mortality. Major gaps in people knowledge of the origin, epidemiology, duration of human transmission and clinical spectrum of disease need fulfilment by future studies.

48. Genomic Characterisation and Epidemiology of 2019 Novel Coronavirus

In late Dec., 2019, patients presenting with viral pneumonia because of an unidentified microbial agent were reported in Wuhan, China. A CoV was identified as the causative pathogen: SARS-CoV-2. As of Jan. 26, 2020, more than 2000 cases of SARS-CoV-2 infection were confirmed, most of which involved people living in or visiting Wuhan, and human-to-human transmission was confirmed. The NGS of samples from bronchoalveolar lavage fluid and cultured isolates from nine inpatients, eight of whom visited the Huanan seafood market in Wuhan were done [54]. Complete and partial SARS-CoV-2 genome sequences were obtained from the individuals. Viral contigs were connected *via* Sanger sequencing to obtain the full-length genomes, with the terminal regions determined by rapid amplification of complementary deoxyribonucleic acid ends. Phylogenetic analysis of SARS-CoV-2 genomes and other CoVs was used to determine the evolutionary history of the virus and help infer its likely origin. Homology modelling was done to explore the likely receptor-binding properties of the virus. The SARS-CoV-2 is sufficiently divergent from SARS-CoV to be considered a new human-infecting β-CoV. Although the phylogenetic analysis suggests that bats might be the original host of the virus, an animal sold at the seafood market in Wuhan might represent an intermediate host facilitating the emergence of the virus in humans. Structural analysis suggests that SARS-CoV-2 might be able to bind to ACE2 receptor in humans. The future evolution, adaptation and spread of this virus warrant urgent investigation.

49. Design and Discovery of Anti-CoV Drugs via Molecular Modelling

With reference to ongoing chaos caused by CoV globally, an urgent need exists to identify a drug, which can inhibit the binding and replication of the virus in humans. In the wake of the emergency situation, if a researcher has any designed compounds, which he thinks might act *vs.* CoV, he can avail Innovative Informatica Technologies' Computational Drug Discovery Services in specific to fight *vs.* CoV. A sample MM and docking report was published: MM and docking studies of DTQ, THQ, THY, TQ compounds compared with HCQ targeting RBD of SARS-CoV-2 drug target towards finding their potential to act as anti-CoV drug-like small molecule [55]. They are screening compounds *vs.* CoV for the following drug targets: human ACE2 (hACE2), papain-like protease (PL pro), 3C-like protease (3CL pro), RNA-dependent RNA polymerase (RdRp), helicase N7 methyltransferase human dipeptidyl peptidase IV (DDP4), RBD and protease cathepsin L type II transmembrane serine protease (TMPRSS2).

50. Etiology of Epidemic Outbreaks COVID-19 in Wuhan, Hubei, China

Results of analysis of phylogenetic, virological, epidemiological, ecological, clinical data of COVID-19 outbreaks in Wuhan, China in comparison with SARS-2002 and MERS-2012 outbreaks allow the following conclusions [56]. 1) The etiological agent of COVID-19 is

SARS-CoV-2, phylogenetically close to SARS-CoV, isolated from human, and SARS-related viruses isolated from bats (SARS-related bat CoVs), which viruses belong to *Sarbecovirus* subgenus, *Betacoronavirus* genus, *Orthocoronavirinae* subfamily, *Coronaviridae* family (*Cornidovirinea: Nidovirales*). The COVID-19 is a variant of SARS-2002 and is different from MERS-2012 outbreak, which were caused by CoV belonged to the subgenus *Merbecovirus* of the same genus. 2) According to the results of phylogenetic analysis of 35 different β-CoVs, isolated from human and wild animals in 2002–2019, the natural source of COVID-19 and SARS-CoV is bats of *Rhinolophus* genus (*Rhinolophidae*) and, probably, some species of other genera. An additional reservoir of the virus could be an intermediate animal species (snakes, civet, hedgehogs, badgers, *etc.*) that are infected by eating of infected bats. The SARS-like coronaviruses circulated in bats in the interepidemic period (2003–2019). 3) Seasonal CoVs (subgenus *Duvinacovirus*, *Alphacoronavirus*) are currently circulating (Nov. 2019–Jan. 2020) in European, Urals, Siberia and Far East of Russia, along with the influenza viruses A(H1N1)pdm09, A(H3N2) and B, and six other respiratory viruses (HPIV, HAdV, HRSV, HRV, HBoV, HMPV).

51. Do Not Touch: Science against Disinformation in the COVID-19 Pademic

The true role of scientific spreading in CoV fight is to explain the reasons for the recommendations that exist, which is scientific disseminator's role, each one from his knowledge parcel [57]. From chemistry and biochemistry, to explain the why of things, because when one understands why he must follow a recommendation, he assumes it, he understands that it is more important and he is more likely to comply with it regardless of it be an order. What CoV fight can give people is a lesson on how to work in science in a different way, in the sense of sharing, because one of the things to criticize about the science system is that it results quite well built but presents a great imperfection: it is quite opaque. When one does a scientific study, he must pass the peer review, that a magazine accept it, that he publish it, and to be able to access the data you even must be subscribed or pay to that journal; i.e., not everything is freely accessible, and that slows everything down a lot. Negative results are not, but only successes are published, and from what does not work one can learn a lot. Now people are sharing everything. Even studies are published that conclude that a drug is not worth, when three months ago it would not be published, and perhaps 20 other research centres could exist wasting time to reach the same conclusion. It seems fundamental that, in the science system, that reflection be made. The system must change, because it cannot be so parasitized by scientific journals.

52. Ethics and COVID-19: Resource Allocation and Priority-Setting

The conclusions about the fair allocation of scarce resources in countries during COVID-19 outbreak follow [58]. 1) The HC workers and first responders can justifiably be prioritized when allocating some resources because of their contribution to the health and well-being of the community. Their health helps preserve the health of others. 2) Participants of research aimed at developing vaccines, therapies or other critical resources should receive priority in receiving the resources because they have helped save others by their participation. This is not an absolute priority. 3) While the principle of first come, first served is usually applied when allocating resources in HC settings, it is rarely appropriate in an emergency. In practice, it is likely to favour certain groups. 4) Younger populations appear to be at lower risk in COVID-19 context. Consequently, the principle of youngest first should have low priority for vaccine, but perhaps may have more weight if they do become sick and need critical care resources. 5) The allocation of different resources may find ethical justification in different principles or values. 6) Maximizing utility must be balanced with the principle of priority to the worst-off: Centralizing the availability of resources in larger centres may extend their benefits to more people, but may exclude isolated populations and challenge people's concern for those at highest risk.

53. Offline: A Global Health Crisis? No, Something Far Worse

Some clues will be found in Fassin's *Life: A Critical User's Manual* [59]. People must say that it is their task to uncover the biographies of those who lived and died with COVID-19 [60]. It is people's task to resist the biologicalisation of the disease, and instead insist on a COVID-19 social and political critique. It is people's task to understand what the disease means to the lives of those it afflicted and use that understanding not only to change their perspective on the world but also to change the world itself. As Fassin concludes, people's *critique does not have to choose between militancy and lucidity.*

54. Navigating the Clean Energy Transition in the COVID-19 Crisis

What does COVID-19 crisis imply for the energy transition required to keep global warming at bay? Many commentators and advocates were quick to provide answers and ready-made solutions. A step back was taken and a different approach, pursued [61]. Structuring the challenges that arise in different time horizons and offering guiding principles for responses are most useful at the stage. Principles were recommended. 1) Avoid overreacting in the short term. 2) Make use of opportunities for the energy transition in the mid-term. 3) Develop policy designs that could withstand future shocks. While the policy attention is rightfully focused on PH crisis and mitigating its immediate effects, it is important to navigate the situation without jeopardizing the imperative clean energy transition.

55. Epidemiological and Clinical Characteristics of 99 Cases of SARS-CoV-2

In Dec., 2019, a pneumonia associated with SARS-CoV-2 emerged in Wuhan, China. The epidemiological and clinical characteristics of SARS-CoV-2 pneumonia were clarified [62]. All confirmed SARS-CoV-2 cases in Wuhan Jinyintan Hospital in Jan. 1–20, 2020 were included in the retrospective, single-centre study. Cases were confirmed by RT-PCR and were analysed for epidemiological, demographic, clinical and radiological features, and laboratory data. Outcomes were followed up until Jan 25, 2020. Infection of SARS-CoV-2 was of clustering onset, is more likely to affect older males with comorbidities, and can result in severe and even fatal respiratory diseases, e.g., ARDS. Characteristics of patients who died were in line with the MuLBSTA score, an early warning model for predicting mortality in viral pneumonia.

56. SARS-CoV-2 Isolation and Rapid Sharing from First Patient in Australia

The objective was to describe the first SARS-CoV-2 isolation and sequencing in Australia, and rapid sharing of the isolate [63]. The SARS-CoV-2 was isolated from a 58-year-old man from Wuhan, China who arrived in Melbourne on Jan. 19, 2020 and was admitted to Monash Medical Centre, Melbourne from the emergency department on Jan. 24, 2020 with fever, cough and progressive dyspnoea. Outcomes were clinical course and laboratory features of the first reported case of COVID-19 in Australia; isolation, whole genome sequencing, imaging and rapid sharing of virus from the patient. The ability to identify, propagate and internationally share rapidly SARS-CoV-2 isolate is an important step in collaborative scientific efforts to deal effectively with the international PH emergency by developing better diagnostic procedures, vaccine candidates and antiviral agents.

57. European Response to COVID-19: Regulatory Emulation and Coordination

Because of its borderless nature, COVID-19 is a matter of common European interest since its first detection on Europe [64]. The pandemic outbreak was largely handled as an essentially national matter. Member States (MSs) adopted their own different, uncoordinated and competing national responses according to their distinctive risk analysis frameworks, with little regard for the scientific and management advice provided by EU, notably its dedicated legal framework for action on cross-border health threats. To justify such an outcome as the inevitable consequence of EU's limited competence in PH is a well-rehearsed yet largely inaccurate argument, which calls for closer scrutiny.

58. Coronavirus Infections: More Than Just the Common Cold

While the trajectory of the outbreak is impossible to predict, effective response requires prompt action from the standpoint of classic PH strategies to the timely development and implementation of effective countermeasures [65]. The emergence of yet another outbreak of human disease caused by a pathogen from a viral family formerly thought to be relatively benign underscores the perpetual challenge of emerging infectious diseases and the importance of sustained preparedness.

59. Association of Public Health Interventions with COVID-19 Epidemiology

The COVID-19 became a pandemic, and it is unknown if a combination of PH interventions can improve control of the outbreak. The objective is to evaluate the association of PH interventions with the epidemiological features of COVID-19 outbreak in Wuhan, by five periods, according to key events and interventions. In a cohort study, individual-level data on 32 583 laboratory-confirmed COVID-19 cases reported in Dec. 8, 2019–Mar. 8, 2020, were extracted from the municipal Notifiable Disease Report System (e.g., patients' age, sex, residential location, occupation, severity classification) [66]. Exposures were nonpharmaceutical PH interventions (e.g., *cordons sanitaire*, traffic restriction, *social distancing*, home confinement, centralized quarantine, universal symptom survey). Rates of laboratory-confirmed COVID-19 infections, across age, sex and geographic locations were calculated across five periods: Dec. 8–Jan. 9 (no intervention), Jan. 10–22 (massive human movement because of Chinese New Year holiday), Jan. 23–Feb. 1 (*cordons sanitaire*, traffic restriction, home quarantine), Feb. 2–16 (centralized quarantine, treatment) and Feb. 17–Mar. 8 (universal symptom survey). The effective reproduction number R_t of SARS-CoV-2 (an indicator of secondary transmission) was calculated over the periods. A series of multifaceted PH interventions was temporally associated with improved control of COVID-19 outbreak in Wuhan, China. The findings may inform PH policy in other countries and regions. The US Centers for Disease Control and Prevention (CDC) must regularly report on R_t for US and each of 50 states, so that political and PH leaders can gauge how well the combined organizational and individual *social distancing* measures in place around the country are working to diminish transmission of the virus [67]. The CDC must communicate this transparently to the public to increase public buy-in and understanding of the actions being taken to slow COVID-19 spread.

60. Choices for the New Normal

Most important of all: Is this the time for equity, when the evidence of global interconnectedness and the vulnerabilities of marginalized people will catalyze at last the fair and compassionate redistribution of wealth, security and opportunity from the few, and fortunate to the rest (*cf.* Figure 12) [68]? The virus awaits an answer. So will the next one.

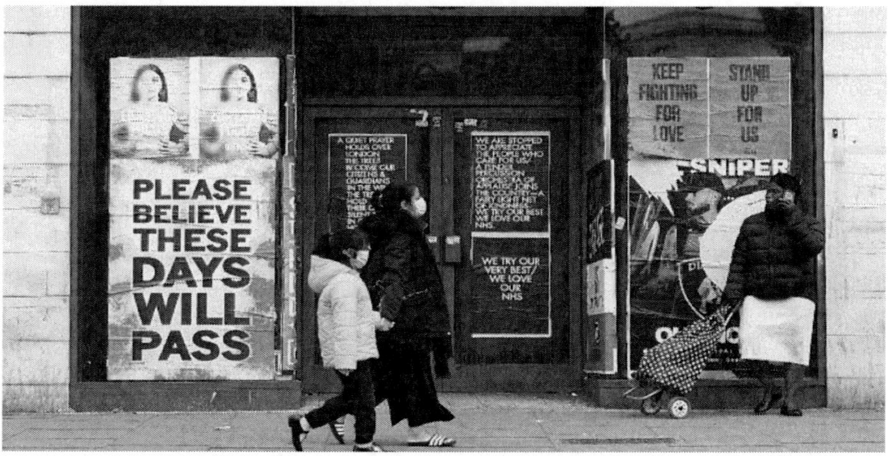
PLEASE BELIEVE THESE DAYS WILL PASS
WE TRY OUR VERY BEST/ WE LOVE OUR NHS
KEEP FIGHTING FOR LOVE
STAND UP FOR US
SNIPER

Figure 12. Please believe these days will pass. Source: RTVE.

61. COVID-19: Remaking the Social Contract

In spite of important deficiencies in some responses, in many ways the world is witnessing the setting aside of ideology to address the urgent and fundamental need common to all people (protection of health) [69]. The taken measures were uneven, short-term and reactive. However, it is hard to imagine that when the pandemic is over, the public will be content to go back to the way things were. It toke a crisis of this scale to force the recognition that the basic role of a government is to serve and protect its people (that wellbeing has a higher value than gross domestic product) is a shocking demonstration of how the reciprocal rights and responsibilities that form the basis of so many democratic systems were hollowed out. The kind of societies that are set to emerge from the pandemic is far from clear, but people's interconnectedness and interdependence at local, national and global levels were never more undeniable. Nor can the importance of well-resourced and -prepared health systems continue to be ignored. A renewed and expanded social contract, one with health at the centre, could well be one legacy of COVID-19.

62. COVID-19 Puts Societies to the Test

The potential fallout of an economic downturn on physical and mental health are likely to be profound but they are not inevitable [70]. Identifying and ensuring that the most at risk are protected, government measures will be crucial in mitigating widening inequalities and PH consequences. For Amartya Sen, writing in *The Financial Times* on Apr. 15, 2019 about the policies enacted so far, *equity has not been a particularly noticeable priority*, still a better society can emerge from the lockdowns. The world paused (an opportunity exists to invest in social protection, prioritise policies to reduce inequalities, give equity a particularly noticeable priority).

63. Community Particiapation Is Crucial in a Pandemic

Institutional cultures that support coproduction must be created in political and health systems [71]. Mechanisms to ensure citizen participation are essential for high-quality, inclusive disaster response and preparedness, which can be called upon again in future emergencies. All societies present community groups that could co-create better pandemic response and health services, and politicians must be supported to incorporate the voices. Such public participation will reveal policy gaps and the potential negative consequences of any response (and identify ways to address these together). Community participation holds the promise of reducing immediate damage from COVID-19 pandemic and, crucially, of building future resilience.

64. Managing Disasters Amid COVID-19 Pandemic: Flood-Disaster Response

The world faces difficulties managing disasters while making efforts to slowing COVID-19 spread. A report aimed at proposing policies and approaches to manage dual disasters of flooding and COVID-19 [72]. It reviewed on-going efforts of organizations in the humanitarian assistance, water and sanitation, disaster management and health sectors. Based on review works, the policy was recommended. The objective of the policy is to protect human life, in particular, vulnerable groups, from the human security perspective. Local organizations and communities play an important role in disaster management, and risk information supported by scientific knowledge is essential. As the experience of disaster management shows, a number of organizations (e.g., health, water) must be coordinated to conduct measures.

65. Quantifying SARS-CoV-2 Transmission Suggests Digital Contact Tracing

The emergent human virus SARS-CoV-2 results in high fatality rates and incapacitated health systems. Preventing further transmission is a priority. Key parameters of epidemic spread were analyzed to estimate the contribution of different transmission routes, and determine requirements for case isolation and contact-tracing needed to stop the epidemic [73]. Viral spread is too fast to be contained by manual contact tracing, but could be controlled if the process were faster, more efficient and happened at scale. A contact-tracing App, which builds a memory of proximity contacts and immediately notifies contacts of positive cases, can achieve epidemic control if used by enough people. Targeting recommendations to only those at risk, epidemics could be contained without need for mass quarantines (*lock-downs*) that are harmful to society. The ethical requirements for an intervention of this kind were discussed.

66. Estimates of the Severity of CoV Disease 2019: A Model-Based Analysis

Physical function declines in old age, portending disability, increased health expenditures and mortality. Cellular senescence, leading to tissue dysfunction, may contribute to the consequences of ageing, but if senescence can directly drive age-related pathology and be therapeutically targeted is still unclear. A study showed that transplanting relatively small numbers of senescent cells into young mice is sufficient to cause persistent physical dysfunction and spread cellular senescence to host tissues [74]. Transplanting even fewer senescent cells had the same effect in older recipients and was accompanied by reduced survival, indicating the potency of senescent cells in shortening health- and lifespan. The senolytic cocktail, dasatinib plus quercetin, which causes selective elimination of senescent cells, decreased the number of naturally occurring senescent cells and their secretion of frailty-related proinflammatory cytokines in explants of human adipose tissue. Intermittent oral administration of senolytics to senescent cell–transplanted young and naturally aged mice alleviated physical dysfunction and increased post-treatment survival by 36%, while reducing mortality hazard to 65%. The study provided proof-of-concept evidence that senescent cells could cause physical dysfunction and decreased survival even in young mice, while senolytics can enhance remaining health- and lifespan in old mice.

In the face of rapidly changing data, a range of case fatality ratio estimates for COVID-19 were produced that differ substantially in magnitude. A study provided robust estimates, accounting for censoring and ascertainment biases [75]. Individual-case data were collected for patients who died from COVID-19 in Hubei, mainland China (reported by national, provincial health commissions to Feb. 8, 2020), and cases outside of mainland China (from government or ministry of health websites, media reports for 37 countries, Hong Kong, Macau, until Feb. 25, 2020), which were used to estimate the time between symptoms onset and outcome (death, discharge from hospital). Age-stratified estimates of the case fatality ratio were obtained relating the aggregate distribution of cases to the observed cumulative deaths in China, assuming a constant attack rate by age, and adjusting for demography, and age-based and location-based under-ascertainment. The case fatality ratio from individual line-list data were estimated on 1 334 cases identified outside of mainland China. *Via* data on the prevalence of PCR-confirmed cases in international residents repatriated from China, age-stratified estimates of the infection fatality ratio were obtained. Data on age-stratified severity in a subset of 3 665 cases from China were used to estimate the proportion of infected individuals who are likely to require hospitalisation. The early estimates give an indication of the fatality ratio across COVID-19 spectrum and show a strong age gradient in risk of death. The overall death rate from COVID-19 was estimated at 0.66%, rising sharply to 7.8% in people aged over 80 and decaying to 0.0016% in children aged nine and under [76].

67. Understanding Coronavirus

Since the identification of the first CoV cases in Dec. 2019 in Wuhan, China, a significant amount of confusion existed regarding SARS-CoV-2 (*coronavirus*) origin and spread, and COVID-19 cause [77].

Conflicting messages from the media and officials across different countries and organizations, the abundance of disparate sources of information, unfounded conspiracy theories on the origins of the emerging virus and the inconsistent PH measures across different countries, all served to increase the level of anxiety in the population. Where did the virus come from? How is it transmitted? How does it cause disease? Is it like flu? What is a pandemic? What can one do to stop its spread? The concise and accessible introduction provides answers to the most common questions surrounding coronavirus for a general audience.

68. The Equitable Distribution of COVID-19 Therapautics and Vaccines

If nations pursue a competitive race to develop effective vaccines and therapeutics, only losers, no winners will exist [78]. Threat of COVID-19 knows no borders. Only a well-coordinated global plan that harnesses the best science and delivers it to everyone in need can effectively counteract the COVID-19 scourge and future pandemics.

69. The COVID-19 Virus Was Neither Created Nor Escaped from a Laboratory

Science came a long way in the few months of a pandemic [79]. Genomes of SARS-CoV-2 were sequenced, and already thousands of virus sequences obtained in many countries exist. Information flows almost in RT. If evidence exists that SARS-CoV-2 is a tampered virus, why has not the evidence that Luc Montagnier talks about in his interview been published? In this way, the scientific community could comment. Meanwhile, the evidences are what they are.

70. THE ORIGIN OF THE SARS-COV-2 CORONAVIRUS, IN LIGHT OF EVOLUTION

Anthropocene humanity faces fabulous challenges (e.g., climate crisis, diseases emergence) that, boarded by airplanes, rapidly globalize [80]. As Rees states, people have nowhere to hide if a pandemic, or collapse economic or in food supply exists [81]. To meet the challenges, people need to rethink many aspects of their daily lives, scales of values, economic and cultural practices; in short, their coexistence with the rest of nature and, especially, their respect for non-human animals. Life is promiscuous, which shaped biodiversity throughout evolution, e.g., humans. However, people's responsibility as a conscious species is to prevent the promiscuity's dark side from causing avoidable harm and pain. People must learn from COVID-19 pandemic to anticipate the next zoonosis that could be even more devastating. In 18th century, Hume and Laplace taught people that extraordinary claims require extraordinary proof [82]. Faced with claims of an SARS-CoV-2's artificial origin or a leak from Wuhan laboratory, its authors provide no evidence. Not even ordinary. Let people not give the fake news any credit and focus on what science says, because only research in the fields of virology, genetics and evolution will allow knowing how the virus originated, which will contribute decisively to the development of drugs and vaccines, with which people will finally succeed in overcoming COVID-19 pandemic.

71. THIS IS WHAT VIROLOGISTS KNOW TO DATE ABOUT SARS-COV-2 CORONAVIRUS

Let people not forget that, according to a study by researchers from Boston School of Public Health published in the journal *Science*, even in the case of the apparent elimination of the pandemic in the coming months, the estimates for the post-pandemic periods foresee occasional outbreaks until 2024 [83]. People have no choice but to be prepared.

72. University Teachers Mutation/Extinction in Digital Age: Adapt or Die

The university professor is obliged to move to a techno-digital profile in which he integrate his current competences with the digital ones [84]. Those who do not adapt to this will be functional illiterates and will be vulnerable to extinction. Digital skills will be essential for future teaching because young people are digital. Let people hope that personnel selection in the future take into account the digital aspect of the teacher, not only the academic, research and management aspects; i.e., that the digital footprint be taken into account and that professionals be valued as teachers from this perspective, not only in terms of their online profile but also in connection with the sector, their position as a researcher and positioning of their research [85]. The absence of a digital brand will be an indication of the absence of digital skills, essential for a teacher in 21st century.

73. University Must Be Renewed in a Virtual Environment without Losing Essence

Virtuality is fertile ground, even for the emergence of occurrences that squander the ends of university education [86]. People will have to be vigilant because everything indicates that more ingenuities will come. In addition, people will have to think if they improve university education or do it a disservice, if they make people something else or allow people to continue being a community of explorers of knowledge, truth, beauty and goodness. In addition, in virtuality.

74. Educating in Times of Confinement: Task of Renewing a Common World

The balance could not be more positive, given the commitment with which the various educational agents know how to face the difficult situation that the pandemic opened for people [87]. However, it leads people to make a wake-up call on educational and social inequality, and the consequences that the crisis has and will have from the transversal inequality perspective [88].

75. COVID-19: Pandemic of Mathematical Models

People are in the descent of the contagion curve, but they are in the ascending phase of predictive models [89]. Every day models appear, whose predictions seem to be subject to contagion, since it is shocking that with such a degree of uncertainty so much consensus exists in the results between models. Time will tell. For now, it is time to thank the efforts of the scientific modelling community to shine the crystal ball. Models can be run online. Let people be optimistic: scientific collaboration, sharing open source models, e.g., EpiNow (in R), and available resource libraries for modelling COVID-19 will provide useful information for making sound decisions.

76. Not All Data Are the Same: Context in Pandemic Information

Regardless of the figures, the lessons learned are fundamental, to the extent that people be able to accumulate experience and extract knowledge from COVID-19-produced data, incorporate them into collective intelligence [90]. To distill learning, it is necessary to analyze the contexts in which the pandemic develops and the factors that explain its causes and consequences.

77. Clinical Characteristics of the Recovered COVID-19 Patients

A large study in SK confirms that in 260 studied cases, only dead parts of the virus were detected. The UK placed Ab tests, which check if someone had Covid-19, at the centre of an eventual *back-to-work* plan to restart normal life. However, experts said they may not prove if someone is protected from reinfection. The UK's testing co-ordinator warned people not to buy private tests. Some infections present a lifelong immunity after being overcome; others, temporary protection; others, none at all. In CoV case, no certainties exist. The alleged cases of reinfected patients in SK after passing COVID-19 turned out to be *false positives*, as reported by SK's health authorities. The news alleviates the fear that no immunity to the coronavirus exists after overcoming the disease. Cases recovered from COVID-19 tested positive for SARS-CoV-2 after discharge (re-detectable positive, RP); however RP-patients clinical characteristics, significance and potential cause remained elusive. A total of 262 COVID-19 patients were discharged in Jan. 23–Feb. 25, 2020, and were enrolled for analysis of their clinical parameters [91]. The RP and non-RP (NRP) patients were grouped according to the disease severity during their hospitalization period. The clinical characterization at re-admission to the hospital was analyzed. The SARS-CoV-2 RNA and plasma Ab levels were detected *via* high-sensitive detection methods. Young and mild COVID-19 patients seem to be RP patients after discharge, who show no obviously clinical symptoms and disease progression upon re-admission. More sensitive RNA detection methods are required to monitor the patients during follow-up. The findings provide empirical information and evidence for the effective management of COVID-19 patients during convalescent phase.

78. Good Practices in the Work Centres: Prevention of COVID-19 Contagions

Organizational measures follow [92]. 1) In accordance with the regulations on occupational risks, it will be necessary to inform the staff in a reliable, updated and habitual way of the health recommendations that they must follow individually. 2) It is necessary to provide the personnel with the necessary hygiene products to be able to follow the individual recommendations, adapting to each specific activity. In general, it is necessary to maintain an adequate supply of soap, hydroalcoholic solution and disposable tissues. 3) A sufficient supply of cleaning materials must be maintained to be able to undertake reinforced sanitation tasks on a daily basis; e.g., bleach and products authorized by the Ministry of Health to disinfect. 4) It is necessary to have a sufficient supply of protection material, especially gloves and masks, for personnel when indicated by the occupational risk prevention service and, specifically, the most exposed (company doctors and nurses, cleaning personnel, staff facing the public). 5) Specific measures must be adopted to minimize the risk of transmission to especially sensitive workers when they must go to the workplace. 6) It is advisable to carry out a contingency plan, identifying the risk of exposure to the virus from the different activities carried out in the workplace, adopting protection measures in each case in accordance with the applicable regulations at all times. For the elaboration of the plan, prevention delegates or workers' representatives must be consulted. 7) It is necessary to establish protocols in the event that a working person manifests symptoms in their workplace, to protect them and protect the rest of the workforce [follow recommendations Procedure for occupational risk prevention services against exposure to SARS-CoV-2 (COVID19) of the Ministry of Health] [93].

79. COVID-19 Arrival in a Context of Climate Emergency: A Crisis of Crises

After Bassett and Fogelman, it is especially interesting to apply an analysis from the perspective of political ecology to examine social, political and economic processes at various scales that shape vulnerabilities and opportunities to overcome adversity. At the very least, the recommendations are intended to avoid the risk of turning sustainable adaptation into an oxymoron [94], a danger that was warned by environmental social scientists, e.g., Katrina Brown.

80. Gender and COVID-19: Advocacy Brief

The WHO's advocacy brief on gender and COVID-19 concluded [95]: 1) The MSs and partners are encouraged to collect, report and analyse data on confirmed COVID-19 cases and deaths that be disaggregated by sex and age, at a minimum, in accordance with WHO's global surveillance and national surveillance guidance. The MSs are urged to conduct a gender data analysis, and invest in quality gender-responsive research on the potentially differential adverse health, social and economic impacts of COVID-19 on women and men. The findings of such analysis must be used to fine-tune response policies. 2) The MSs and partners are encouraged to include responses to violence *vs.* women, and particularly intimate partner violence, as an essential service in COVID-19 response, resource this adequately and identify ways of making services accessible in lockdown-measures context. 3) The MSs and partners are encouraged to maintain the availability of, and equitable access to, sexual and reproductive health services, and include them in the essential package of health services for COVID-19 response. 4) The MSs and partners are encouraged to ensure that all front-line health, and social workers and caregivers have equitable access to training, PPE and other essential products, psychosocial support and social protection, taking into account the specific needs of women who constitute the majority of such workers. 5) The MSs and partners are encouraged to remove financial and other barriers to COVID-19 testing and treatment services, making them free at the point of use. Equitable access to essential health services, and access to safe water and sanitation facilities, must be ensured in disadvantaged areas (e.g., rural communities, informal settlements). Safety nets to mitigate the adverse and inequitable social and economic impacts of the pandemic (e.g., sick leave, unemployment benefits) must be ensured to support containment measures. 6) The MSs and partners are encouraged to stress that health be a human right, to ensure that emergency COVID-19 responses be inclusive and nondiscriminatory, and avoid excessive use of emergency powers to regulate day-to-day life. Such powers must never be used indefinitely but solely with a view to facilitating a return to normal life. The MSs must take measures to identify and counter stigmatizing and discriminatory practices in COVID-19 responses.

81. Severe COVID-19: Recent Progress with a Look towards the Future

Strained HC systems, lockdowns and safety requirements hampered efforts to collect tissue from patients that is crucial to research [96]. The COVID-19 is an acute infectious disease caused by SARS-CoV-2 infection. The WHO confirmed that COVID-19 is a global infectious disease pandemic, which is the third acute infectious disease caused by CoV infection in 21st century, after SARS/MERS. Damage mechanism of SARS-CoV-2 is unclear: It is possible that protein S bind to ACE2 receptors and invade alveolar epithelial cells, causing direct toxic effects and an excessive immune response, which stimulates a systemic inflammatory response, forming a cytokine storm, which leads to lung tissue injury. In severe cases, the disease can lead to ARDS, septic shock, metabolic acidosis, coagulation dysfunction and multiple organ dysfunction syndromes. Severe-COVID-19 patients present a relatively high mortality rate. Currently, no specific antiviral drugs exist for COVID-19 treatment. Most patients need to be admitted to ITU for intensive monitoring and supportive organ function treatments. Severe-COVID-19 epidemiology, pathogenesis, clinical manifestations, diagnosis and treatment methods were reviewed, and tentative ideas were put forward, aiming to provide guidance for severe-COVID-19 diagnosis and treatment [97].

82. Evolutionary-Epidemiological Model for an Asymptomatic Infection

Pathogens exhibit a rich variety of life history strategies, shaped by natural selection. An important pathogen life history characteristic is the propensity to induce an asymptomatic yet productive (transmissive) stage at the beginning of an infection, which characteristic is subject to complex trade-offs, ranging from immunological considerations to population-level social processes. The evolutionary dynamics of such asymptomatic pathogens behaviour (*latency*) was classified, in order to unify epidemiology and evolution for the life history strategy [98]. The focus was on a simple epidemiological model with two infectious stages, where hosts in the first stage can be partially or fully asymptomatic. Immunologically, a trade-off exists between transmission and progression in this first stage. For arbitrary trade-offs, different conditions were derived that guarantee either at least one evolutionarily stable strategy at zero, some or maximal latency of the first stage, or, perhaps surprisingly, at least one unstable evolutionarily singular strategy. In the latter, bistability exists between zero and nonzero (possibly maximal) latency. The uniqueness of interior evolutionarily singular strategies for power-law and exponential trade-offs were proved: Bistability is always between zero and maximal latency. Overall, previous multistage infection models can be summarized with a single model that includes evolutionary processes acting on latency. Since small changes in parameter values can lead to abrupt transitions in evolutionary dynamics, appropriate disease control strategies could have a substantial impact on the evolution of first-stage latency.

83. Airborne Lifetime of Small Speech Droplets in SARS-CoV-2 Transmission

Speech droplets generated by asymptomatic SARS-CoV-2 carriers are increasingly considered to be a likely mode of disease transmission [99]. Highly sensitive laser light scattering observations revealed that loud speech could emit thousands of oral fluid droplets per second. In a closed, stagnant air environment, they disappear from the window of view with time constants in 8–14 min, which corresponds to droplet nuclei of 4 μm diameter, or 12–21-μm droplets before dehydration, which observations confirm that a substantial probability exists that normal speaking cause airborne virus transmission in confined environments.

84. A Bat CoV Related to SARS-CoV-2 Contains Insertions in the Spike Protein

The unprecedented pandemic of SARS-CoV-2-caused pneumonia in China and beyond had major PH impacts on a global scale. Although bats are the most likely natural hosts for SARS-CoV-2, virus origins remain unclear. A bat-derived CoV (RmYN02) identified from a metagenomic analysis of samples from 227 bats collected from Yunnan Province (China) in May–Oct. 2019 was reported [100]. The RmYN02 shares 93.3% nucleotide identity with SARS-CoV-2 at the scale of the complete virus genome and 97.2% identity in the 1ab gene, in which it is the closest SARS-CoV-2 relative reported to date. In contrast, RmYN02 showed low sequence identity (61.3%) to SARS-CoV-2 in RBD and might not bind to ACE2. Critically, and in a similar manner to SARS-CoV-2, RmYN02 was characterized by the insertion of multiple amino acids (AAs) at the junction site of S1 and S2 subunits of the spike (S) protein, which provides strong evidence that such insertion events could occur naturally in animal β-CoVs.

85. Are Pangolins the Intermediate Host of the 2019 Novel SARS-CoV-2?

Outbreak of COVID-19 in Wuhan City, China resulted in more than 1 700 000 laboratory confirmed cases all over the world. Studies showed that SARS-CoV-2 was likely originated from bats, but its intermediate hosts are still largely unknown. The complete genome of a CoV identified in three sick Malayan pangolins was assembled [101]. The molecular and phylogenetic analyses showed that the pangolin CoV (pangolin-CoV-2020) is genetically related to SARS-CoV-2 and a group of bat CoV, but do not support SARS-CoV-2 emerged directly from pangolin-CoV-2020. Pangolins are natural hosts of *Betacoronaviruses*. Large surveillance of CoVs in pangolins could improve people's understanding of the spectrum of CoVs in pangolins. In addition to conservation of wildlife, minimizing the exposures of humans to wildlife will be important to reduce the spillover risks of CoVs from wild animals to humans.

86. SARS-CoV-2 Cross-Neutralization by Monoclonal SARS-CoV Antibody

The SARS-CoV-2 is responsible for COVID-19 pandemic, which resulted in 3 700 000 infections and 260 000 deaths as of 6 May 2020. Vaccine and therapeutic discovery efforts are paramount to curb the pandemic spread of the zoonotic virus. The SARS-CoV-2 spike (S) glycoprotein promotes entry into host cells and is the main target of neutralizing Abs. Multiple mAbs targeting SARS-CoV-2 S were described, identified from memory B cells of an individual who was infected with

SARS-CoV in 2003 [102]. One Ab (S309) potently neutralizes SARS-CoV-2 and SARS-CoV pseudoviruses, and authentic SARS-CoV-2 by engaging S RBD. *Via* cryo-EM and binding assays, S309 recognizes a glycan-containing epitope that is conserved within the sarbecovirus subgenus, without competing with receptor attachment. Cocktails of Ab including S309 and other Abs enhanced SARS-CoV-2 neutralization and may limit the emergence of neutralization-escape mutants. The results pave the way for using S309- and S309-containing Ab cocktails for prophylaxis in individuals at high risk of exposure, or as a post-exposure therapy to limit or treat severe disease.

87. Is Photography a Lie?

Universitat of Valencia organized a web seminar on whether photography is a lie (*cf.* Figure 13) [103].

Figure 13. Is photography a lie?

Pandemic of Covid-19 plunged people into a deep crisis, which is not only health but also economic, financial, labour and social. The scenario of radical uncertainty people face affects all areas of human existence and the organization of social life (e.g., artistic, cultural, moral dimensions). A Q was raised.

> Q1. (Ariño). What maneuver does the photojournalist have over the control of his photographs?

88. Lessons from the Pandemic: Test Surfaced Strengths and Weaknesses

Crisis depth goes beyond the demographic, economic or health impact [104]. It affects human relationships and values. The experience must serve to educate citizens in a more rational use of health resources, excessive drug use, hospital emergencies, in short, to highlight caring importance for the common good, PH. Because today, people know that an illness could trigger a great catastrophe, and this global process makes individual responsibility more important and the public good becomes even more valuable.

89. Airway Driving Pressure and Lung Stress in Ards Patients

Lung-protective ventilation strategy suggests the use of low tidal volume, depending on ideal body weight, and adequate levels of positive end-expiratory pressure (PEEP). However, reducing tidal volume according to ideal body weight does not always prevent overstress and overstrain. On the contrary, titrating mechanical ventilation on airway driving pressure, computed as airway pressure changes from PEEP to end-inspiratory plateau pressure, equivalent to the ratio between the tidal volume and compliance of respiratory system, must better reflect lung injury. However, possible changes in chest wall elastance could affect the reliability of airway driving pressure. A study showed that airway driving pressure could accurately predict lung stress (the pressure generated into the lung because of PEEP and tidal volume) [105]. A total of 150 ARDS patients were enrolled. At 5 and 15 cmH_2O of PEEP, lung stress, driving pressure, lung and chest wall elastance were measured. Airway driving pressure can detect lung overstress with an acceptable accuracy.

90. Driving Pressure and Survival in Acute Respiratory Distress Syndrome

Mechanical-ventilation strategies that use lower end-inspiratory (plateau) airway pressures, lower tidal volumes (V_T) and higher PEEPs can improve survival in patients with ARDS, but the relative importance of each component is uncertain. Because respiratory-system compliance (C_{RS}) is strongly related to the volume of aerated remaining functional lung during disease (*functional lung size*), it was hypothesized that driving pressure ($\Delta P = V_T/C_{RS}$), in which V_T is intrinsically normalized to functional lung size (instead of predicted lung size in healthy persons), would be an index more strongly associated with survival than V_T or PEEP in patients who are not actively breathing [106]. *Via* a statistical tool known as multilevel mediation analysis to analyze individual data from 3 562 patients with ARDS enrolled in nine previously reported randomized trials, ΔP was examined as an independent variable associated with survival. In the mediation analysis, the isolated effects of changes in ΔP resulting from randomized ventilator settings were estimated, while minimizing confounding because of the baseline severity of lung disease. The ΔP was the ventilation variable that best stratified risk. Decreases in ΔP because of changes in ventilator settings were strongly associated with increased survival.

91. Lactic Acidosis: An Update

Lactate is one of the most crucial intermediates in carbohydrate and nonessential AA metabolism. The complexity of cellular interactions and metabolism means that lactate can be considered a waste product for one cell, but a useful substrate for another. The presence of elevated lactate levels in critically ill patients presents important implications for morbidity and mortality. Lactate metabolism, lactic-acidosis pathophysiology, D-lactate clinical significance, lactate-measurement role in acutely ill patients, the methods used to measure lactate in blood or plasma, and some methodological issues related to interferences in the assays, especially in ethylene glycol poisoning, were reviewed [107].

92. Extracorporeal Membrane Oxygenation for Severe Ards

Venovenous extracorporeal membrane oxygenation (ECMO) efficacy in severe-ARDS patients remains controversial. In an international CT, severe-ARDS patients were randomly assigned, as indicated by one criterion [a ratio of partial pressure of arterial O_2 (PaO_2) to the fraction of inspired O_2 (FiO_2) of less than 50 mm Hg for more than 3h, a PaO_2:FiO_2 of less than 80 mm Hg for more than 6h or an arterial blood p*H* of less than 7.25 with a partial pressure of arterial CO_2 of at least 60 mm Hg for more than 6h] to receive immediate venovenous ECMO (ECMO group) or continued conventional treatment (control group) [108]. Crossover to ECMO was possible for patients in the control group who had refractory hypoxemia. The primary end point was mortality at 60d. Among severe-ARDS patients, 60-d mortality was not significantly lower with ECMO than a strategy of conventional mechanical ventilation that included ECMO as rescue therapy.

93. Trauma or Personal Growth? Possible Futures after a Pandemic

A study tested a cognitive model of posttraumatic symptoms (PTSs) and growth (PTG) after exposure to a natural disaster [109]. It was hypothesized that although subjective severity of trauma would be related to PTS severity, the relation would be mediated by brooding and cognitive strategies related to the presence of repetitive negative content in thoughts. The severity–PTG relation would be fully mediated by deliberate rumination (DR), cognitive strategies related to conscious efforts focused on handling the event. To evaluate the cognitive model, adults who lost their homes as a result of the earthquake and tsunami that occurred in Chile on Feb. 27, 2010, were selected. Structural equation modelling was used to analyse the data. The resulting model presented adequate indices of goodness adjustment and showed that brooding completely mediated subjective severity–PTS relation, and DR completely mediated subjective severity–brooding–PTG relation, which results highlight the role of rumination content and process in mediating trauma subjective severity–PTS–PTG association. Results implications for a more comprehensive model of symptom severity that occurs after trauma were discussed. In the crisis, suffering exists and will exist [110]. However, surely also growth, because both are not antithetical. Both will teach people to understand better their weaknesses and strengths. As individuals and a nation.

94. What Social Changes Will the Coronavirus Bring People?

On the capacity that people present to respond to the crisis, not only in health, but also in economic and social terms, taking advantage of the positive elements of the ongoing transformations and compensating for the negative ones, depends on the type of society in that they will live in the future [111, 112].

95. Online vs. Classroom Education: There Is No Place Like School to Learn

It depends on all, people and institutions called to responsibly exercise their teaching work [113]. It will be people's task that, after the experience, they continue to claim direct, real interaction as the most appropriate, albeit costly and demanding, way of an educational relationship. People could repeat that they do not value what they have until they lost it. People could have a chance to get it back.

96. Who Is Afraid of the Ferocious Hoax?

If all people are capable of doing in this context is using their experts to discredit ones on the other side, they will be unable to reverse polarization trend [114]. Hoaxes will then be the least of people's problems.

97. Hydroxychloroquine or Chloroquine with or without a Macrolide

The COVID-19 may disproportionately affect people with CVD. Concern was aroused regarding a potential harmful effect of ACE inhibitors and angiotensin-receptor blockers (ARBs) in this clinical context. *Via* an observational database from 169 hospitals in Asia, Europe and North America, CVD–drug therapy relationship was evaluated with in-hospital death among hospitalized COVID-19 patients who were admitted in Dec. 20, 2019–Mar. 15, 2020, and were recorded in Surgical Outcomes Collaborative registry as died in the hospital or survived to discharge as of Mar. 28, 2020 [115]. The study confirmed previous observations suggesting that underlying CVD results associated with an increased risk of in-hospital death among hospitalized COVID-19 patients. The results did not confirm previous concerns regarding a potential harmful association of ACE inhibitors or ARBs with in-hospital death in the clinical context. The HCQ or CQ, usually in combination with a second-generation macrolide, are widely used for COVID-19 treatment, despite no conclusive evidence of their benefit. Although generally safe when used for approved indications (e.g., autoimmune disease, malaria) treatment-regimens safety and benefit are poorly evaluated in COVID-19. A multinational registry analysis of HCQ or CQ use with or without a macrolide for COVID-19 treatment was done [116]. The registry comprised data from 671 hospitals in six continents. Patients hospitalised in Dec. 20, 2019–Apr. 14, 2020, with a positive laboratory finding for SARS-CoV-2 were included. Patients who received one of the treatments of interest within 48h of diagnosis were included in one of four treatment groups (CQ alone, CQ with a macrolide, HCQ alone, HCQ with a macrolide) and patients who received none of the treatments formed the control group. Patients for whom one of the treatments of interest was initiated more than 48h after diagnosis or while they were on mechanical ventilation, and patients who received remdesivir were excluded. The main outcomes of interest were in-hospital mortality and the occurrence of *de-novo* ventricular arrhythmias (non-sustained or sustained ventricular tachycardia, ventricular fibrillation). Benefit of HCQ or CQ, when used alone or with a macrolide, on in-hospital outcomes for COVID-19 was not confirmed. Each drug regimen was associated with decreased in-hospital survival and an increased frequency of ventricular arrhythmias when used for COVID-19 treatment.

98. Modelling Second-Wave Distancing, Testing, Tracing and Quarantine

The COVID-19 required the implementation of severe mobility restrictions and *social distancing* measures worldwide. While the measures were proven effective in abating the epidemic in several countries, it is important to estimate the effectiveness of testing and tracing strategies to avoid a potential second wave of COVID-19 epidemic. Highly detailed (anonymized, privacy-enhanced) mobility data from mobile devices were integrated with census and demographic data to build a detailed agent-based model to describe SARS-CoV-2 transmission dynamics in Boston metropolitan area [117]. Enforcing strict *social distancing* followed by a policy based on a robust level of testing, contact-tracing and household quarantine, could keep the disease at a level that does not exceed HC-system capacity. Assuming the identification of 50% of the symptomatic infections, and the tracing of 40% of their contacts and households, which corresponds to 9% of individuals quarantined, the ensuing reduction in transmission allows economic activities reopening while attaining a manageable impact on HC system. The results show that a response system based on enhanced testing and contact tracing could play a major role in relaxing *social distancing* interventions in the absence of herd immunity *vs*. SARS-CoV-2.

99. Pandemics Meet Democracy: Evidence from COVID-19 Crisis in Spain

Outbreak of COVID-19 poses an unprecedented challenge for contemporary democracies. Despite the global scale of the problem, the response was mainly national, and global coordination was so far extremely weak. All over the world, governments are making use of exceptional powers to enforce lockdowns, usually sacrificing civil liberties and profoundly altering the pre-existing power balance, which nurtures fears of an authoritarian turn. Relief packages to mitigate the economic consequences of the lockdowns are discussed, and little doubt exists that the forthcoming recession will present important distributive consequences. Citizens' responses to the democratic dilemmas were studied [118]. Results from a set of survey experiments run in Spain in Mar. 20–28, 2020 were presented, together with longitudinal evidence from a panel survey fielded right before and after the virus outbreak. The findings reveal a strong preference for a national as opposed to a European/international response. The national bias is much stronger for COVID-19 crisis than for other global problems (e.g., climate change, international terrorism). Widespread demand for strong leadership, willingness to give up individual freedom and a sharp increase in support for technocratic governance were found. As such, the initial switch in mass public preferences towards technocratic and authoritarian government caused by the pandemic was document. To what extent the crisis may contribute to a shift to a self-enforcing political equilibrium was discussed.

100. Behavioural Immune System Is Designed to Avoid Infected Individuals

What is the adapted structure of the behavioural immune system (BIS)? By definition, BIS motivates pathogen avoidance. One prominent suggestion is that BIS contains an additional component that generates motivation to avoid individuals from unfamiliar outgroups. The evolvability of the component was questioned, however, and it was noted that all supportive evidence stems from WEIRD samples. Between-subject experiments were conducted in large samples of adult US and India residents [119]. In the experiment, comfort with physical contact with a depicted individual was measured. The individual was either from an ethnic ingroup or outgroup, and either showed a pathogen cue or not. Results were inconsistent with the view that BIS motivates the avoidance of individuals from unfamiliar outgroups. Instead, the results supported that the system simply motivates the avoidance of any infected individual regardless of their group membership.

101. Targets of T Cell Responses to SARS-CoV-2 in COVID-19 and Unexposed

Understanding adaptive SARS-CoV-2 immunity is important for vaccine development, interpreting COVID-19 pathogenesis and calibration of pandemic control measures. *Via* human leukocyte antigen class I and II, predicted peptide *megapools*, circulating SARS-CoV-2-specific $CD8^+$ and $CD4^+$ T cells were identified in 70 and 100% of COVID-19 convalescent patients, respectively. The $CD4^+$ T cell responses to spike (S), the main target of most vaccine efforts, were robust and correlated with the magnitude of the anti-SARS-CoV-2 immunoglobulin (Ig)G and IgA titers. The M, S and N proteins each accounted for 11–27% of the total $CD4^+$ response, with additional responses commonly targeting nsp3, nsp4, ORF3a, ORF8, *etc*. For $CD8^+$ T cells, S and M were recognized, with at least eight SARS-CoV-2 ORFs targeted. The SARS-CoV-2-reactive $CD4^+$ T cells were detected in 40–60% of unexposed individuals, suggesting cross-reactive T cell recognition between circulating *common cold* CoVs and SARS-CoV-2 (*cf*. Figure 14) [120].

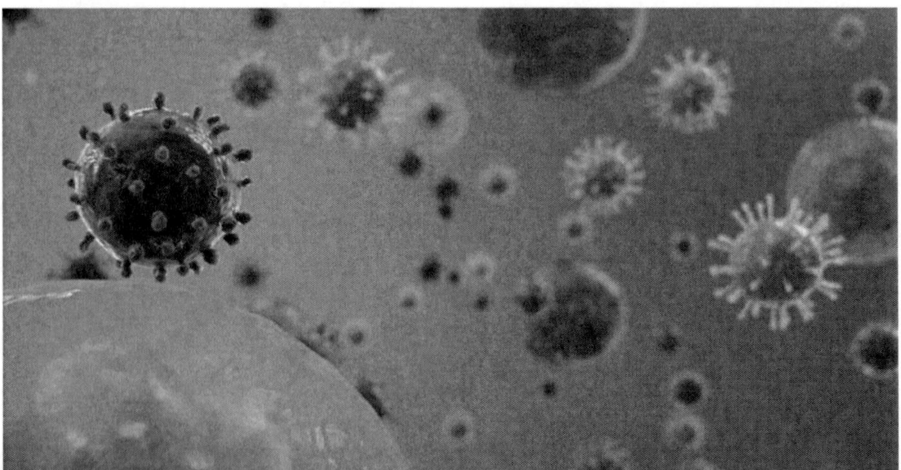

Figure 14. 50% of studied subjects had a significant T-cell reactivity *vs*. SARS-CoV-2. Source: iStock.

102. SARS-CoV-2 Infection Protects against Rechallenge in Rhesus Macaques

An understanding of protective SARS-CoV-2 immunity is critical for vaccine and PH strategies aimed at ending the global COVID-19 pandemic. A question is whether infection with SARS-CoV-2 results in protective immunity *vs.* re-exposure. A rhesus macaque model of SARS-CoV-2 infection was developed, and macaques presented high viral loads in the upper and lower respiratory tract, humoral and cellular immune responses, and pathologic evidence of viral pneumonia [121]. Following initial viral clearance, animals were rechallenged with SARS-CoV-2 and showed 5 $\log_{10}$ reductions in median viral loads in bronchoalveolar lavage and nasal mucosa compared to primary infection. Anamnestic immune responses following rechallenge suggested that protection was mediated by immunologic control. The data show that SARS-CoV-2 infection induced protective immunity *vs.* re-exposure in nonhuman primates.

103. Nurses Know What Went Wrong in Healthcare System

Nurses know what went wrong in HC system: 1) in organization; 2) that the importance of the primary care was not given; 3) many things about an organizational HC system that must be changed to guarantee patient safety (pills, means, organization of the system itself, the ability to supply their own equipment) [122].

Many things exist to consider and they will learn. Others, unfortunately and according to seeing certain empirical behaviours, must learn many more things.

104. Coronavirus: How Biologists Resolved Virus So Spectacularly Quickly

Outbreak of SARS-CoV-2 represents a pandemic threat that was declared an international-concern PH emergency. Spike (S) glycoprotein of CoV is a key target for vaccines, therapeutic Abs and diagnostics. To facilitate medical countermeasure development, a 3.5Å-resolution cryo–EM structure of SARS-CoV-2 S trimer in the prefusion conformation was determined [123]. The predominant state of the trimer presents one of the three RBDs rotated up in a receptor-accessible conformation. The SARS-CoV-2 S protein binds ACE2 with higher affinity than does SARS-CoV S. Published SARS-CoV RBD-specific mAbs were tested and do not present appreciable binding to SARS-CoV-2 S, suggesting that Ab cross-reactivity may be limited between the two RBDs. Structure of SARS-CoV-2 S should enable the rapid development and evaluation of medical countermeasures to address the ongoing PH crisis. Emergence of SARS-CoV-2 resulted in >90 000 infections and >3 000 deaths. Spike (S) glycoproteins of CoV promote entry into cells and are the main Abs target. The SARS-CoV-2 S uses ACE2 to enter cells, and SARS-CoV-2 and SARS-CoV S RBDs bind with similar affinities to human ACE2, correlating with the efficient SARS-CoV-2 spread among humans [124]. The SARS-CoV-2 S glycoprotein harbours a furin cleavage site at the boundary between S_1/S_2 subunits, which is processed during biogenesis and sets the virus apart from SARS-CoV and SARS-related CoVs. Cryo-EM structures of SARS-CoV-2 S ectodomain trimer were determined, providing a blueprint for the design of vaccines and inhibitors of viral entry.

Murine polyclonal Abs of SARS-CoV S potently inhibited SARS-CoV-2 S-mediated entry into cells, indicating that cross-neutralizing Abs targeting conserved S epitopes could be elicited upon vaccination.

105. COVID-19 Survey: How Has COVID-19 Affected One's Academic Life?

T. Deryugina, O. Shurchkov and J. Stearns carried out COVID-19 survey to understand how COVID-19 pandemic is affecting the lives of academics.

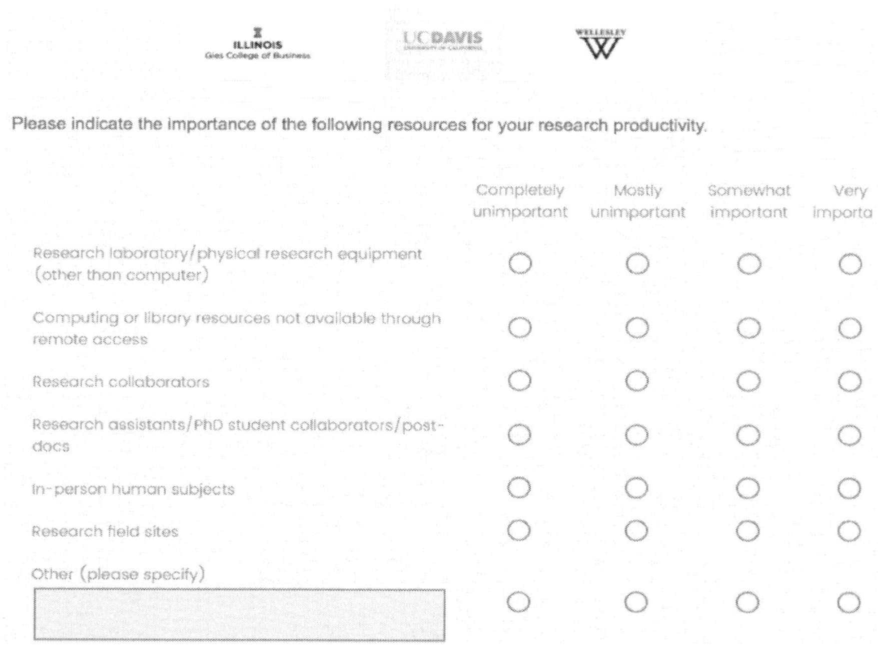

ILLINOIS Gies College of Business UC DAVIS WELLESLEY W

Please indicate the importance of the following resources for your research productivity.

	Completely unimportant	Mostly unimportant	Somewhat important	Very importa
Research laboratory/physical research equipment (other than computer)	○	○	○	○
Computing or library resources not available through remote access	○	○	○	○
Research collaborators	○	○	○	○
Research assistants/PhD student collaborators/post-docs	○	○	○	○
In-person human subjects	○	○	○	○
Research field sites	○	○	○	○
Other (please specify)	○	○	○	○

Figure 15. Survey: Indicate the importance of the following resources for your research productivity.

The research will help inform future institutional and governmental responses to similar shocks. Questions follow.

Q1. Please indicate the importance of the following resources for your research productivity (*cf.* Figure 15).

Completely unimportant Mostly unimportant
Somewhat important Very important
Research laboratory/physical research equipment (other than computer)
Computing or library resources not available *via* remote access
Research collaborators
Research assistants/PhD student collaborators/post-docs
In-person human subjects
Research field sites
Other (please specify)

Q2. To the best of your ability, please estimate the number of HOURS you spend on the activities below on a given WORKDAY both before and after any COVID-19-created disruptions. [Notice that your answers (e.g., the *other* category) must add up to 24 hours, *cf.* Figure 16.]

On average before any COVID-19-created disruptions
On average since any disruptions due to COVID-19
Research
All other job-related activities
Commute to/from work
Childcare and schooling
Housekeeping (cleaning, maintenance, laundry, yardwork, *etc.*)
Sleep
Other
Total 24 24

ILLINOIS Gies College of Business · UC DAVIS · WELLESLEY

To the best of your ability, please estimate the number of HOURS you spend on the activities below on a given WORKDAY both before and after any disruptions created by COVID-19. (Note that your answers -- including the "other" category -- must add up to 24 hours)

	On average prior to any disruptions created by COVID-19	On average since any disruptions due to COVID-19
Research	0	0
All other job-related activities	0	0
Commute to/from work	0	0
Child care and schooling	0	0
Housekeeping (cleaning, maintenance, laundry, yardwork, etc.)	0	0
Sleep	0	0
Other	0	0
Total	0	0

Figure 16. Survey: Estimate the number of hours you spend on activities below on a given workday.

Q3. To the best of your ability, please estimate the number of HOURS your spouse/partner/significant other spends on the activities below on a given WORKDAY both before and after any COVID-19-created disruptions. [Notice that your answers (e.g., the *other* category) must add up to 24 hours.]

On average before any COVID-19-created disruptions
On average since any disruptions due to COVID-19
Work in paid employment
Commute to/from work

Childcare and schooling
Housekeeping (cleaning, maintenance, laundry, yardwork, *etc.*)
Sleep
Other
Total 24 24

Q4. How has your funding for the following expenses been affected by COVID-19?

Significantly increased
Not significantly affected
Significantly reduced
Do not know/not applicable
Research assistance/resources
Teaching assistance/resources
Administrative assistance/resources
Other (please specify)

106. Is COVID-19 Increasingly Benign?

Governments around the world respond to COVID-19 pandemic with unprecedented policies designed to slow the growth rate of infections. Many actions (e.g., closing schools, restricting populations to homes) impose large and visible costs on society, but their benefits cannot be directly observed and are currently understood only *via* process-based simulations. Data were compiled on 1 717 local, regional and national non-pharmaceutical interventions deployed in the ongoing pandemic across localities in China, SK, Italy, Iran, France and US [125]. Reduced-form econometric methods, commonly used to measure the effect of policies on economic growth, were applied to evaluate empirically the effect that the anti-contagion policies had on the growth rate of infections. In the absence of policy actions, early COVID-19 infections exhibit exponential growth rates of 38% per day. Anti-contagion policies significantly and substantially slowed the growth. Policies present different impacts on different populations, but the policy packages now deployed are achieving large, beneficial and measurable health outcomes. Across the six countries, interventions prevented or delayed 62 000 000 confirmed cases, corresponding to averting roughly 530 000 000 total infections, which findings may help inform whether or when the policies must be deployed, intensified or lifted, and can support decision-making in the other 180+ countries where COVID-19 was reported. Research into patients who developed the most severe forms of SARS-CoV-2 infection identified the following severity predictors [126]: 1) advanced age; 2) comorbidities; 3) male sex; 4) genetics; 5) cross-immunity with other coronaviruses; 6) viral inoculum. To prevent damage in future COVID-19 outbreaks, work must be done on the following fronts: 1) improve the health system; 2) protect the most vulnerable, especially the elderly; 3) universalize diagnostic tests so that they can be performed on all and as many times as necessary; 4) consolidate the good habits of *social distancing*, e.g., masks for closed places and with crowds. Facilitating and promoting that the maximum number of people get antibody tests allows knowing how many were exposed and are protected, even if only partially and temporarily. In Madrid, 15% of the population was infected and, even if only for 1–2y, they are protected from reinfection, as a study in macaques showed.

107. Advantages and Disadvantages of Working on-Line for Others

Remote work, in its classic conception of homework as the one that is done outside the usual workplace and without the control of the company, and linked to specific sectors and geographical areas, was overtaken by the reality of a new framework of relationships and a severe impact of new technologies [127]. Nowadays, more than homework, remote and flexible work exists that allows work to be carried out in new environments that do not require the presence of the worker in the workplace. The labour-relations virtualization dissociates or relocates the worker from a specific place and time, which undoubtedly brings with it advantages (e.g., greater flexibility in the management of work time and breaks, reconciliation of working, personal and family life, cost reduction in offices and cost savings on the move, productivity, schedules rationalization, commitment and experience of the employee, attraction and retention of talent, job placement of people with reduced mobility and family responsibilities, absenteeism reduction). However, it also presents drawbacks: data protection, security breaches, techno-stress, continuous hours, computer fatigue, permanent digital connectivity, greater job isolation, loss of corporate identity, deficiencies in face-to-face–remote workers information exchange, transfer of productive-activity costs to the worker without compensation, *etc.* The real impact of work-provision or -organization forms was increased exponentially by COVID-19-pandemic impact, which highlighted their advantages and weaknesses, and the need to address their regulation from a security, certainty and transparency legal framework.

108. The Cruel Pedagogy of the Virus

A world that goes *via* a time of intense transformation requires thinking about its most pressing issues: the multiple ways in which violence is practiced, the unceasing inequality rise, damage to the environment and the beings that inhabit the Earth, human-rights violation, territories militarization or pandemic impact on the social web, especially in its most vulnerable sectors. Far from documenting pessimism, to build theoretical tools to transform situations of injustice into an incessant exercise that links theory with practice is aspired [128].

109. Traffic/Search Engine Analysis in Wuhan Indicates Disease in Fall 2019

The global COVID-19 pandemic was originally linked to a zoonotic spillover event in Wuhan's Huanan Seafood Market in Nov.-Dec., 2019. However, recent evidence suggests that the virus may have already been circulating at the time of the outbreak. Previously validated data streams (satellite imagery of hospital parking lots, Baidu search queries of disease related terms) were used to investigate the possibility [129]. An upward trend was observed in hospital traffic and search volume beginning in late Summer and early Fall 2019. While queries of the respiratory symptom *cough* show seasonal fluctuations coinciding with yearly influenza seasons, *diarrhea* is a more COVID-19 specific symptom and shows an association with the current epidemic. The rise of both precedes the documented start of COVID-19 pandemic in Dec., highlighting the value of novel digital sources for emerging-pathogens surveillance.

110. Homeostasis and Coronavirus Crisis

Homeostasis is the appropriate word [130]. If people's society maintains its internal balances, it is certain that it will survive all crises. Let people make sure that the rope on which they balance is not too loose.

111. Human History Is a Succession of Pandemics but People Do Not Learn

If something changes, let people trust that, among all possible paths, they choose the one that goes *via* science, empathy and sustainability [131]. Let people not turn a virus into a Covid-1984-like Orwellian postpademic.

112. COVID-19 Reminds People That They Are Not Gods (and It Is Good News)

People are *the true architects of their social destiny* [132]. People's worst enemy is themselves, when they think they are arrogant enough to do without others and forget how much they need each other. Hopefully, the crisis will help people *change their way of thinking, feeling and doing*. It would be worth a try. The COVID-19 could eventually make people more human.

113. Bioinformatics Joins the Fight against COVID-19

Crises are said to be, in turn, a source of opportunities [133]. Well, let people hope that the current crisis will serve to reaffirm that the health and experimental sciences must continue to be complemented with the knowledge of computing and statistics in order to solve current and future bioproblems.

114. What Do People Know to Date About the Transmission of SARS-CoV-2?

An example is the study carried out in a hospital in South Africa to resolve a nosocomial outbreak that involved 119 individuals among patients and HC personnel [134]. The really important thing about the type of research is that they are capable of providing valuable information to PH authorities, so that they could adopt measures to control the transmission of the virus.

115. Ten Ideas for a Successful Digital Transit of Universities

Ideas for a successful digital transit of universities follow [135]: 1) justify and explain, with sufficient reasons and plenty of transparency, why people migrate the public university service to an *online* model; 2) clarify what are the competitive advantages that the change of model would offer compared to other institutions; 3) it is not about adding technology to one's university, but applying technology to improve its offerings; 4) are all members of the university sectors trained for change?; 5) people must implement as soon as possible a strategy of digital equity and technology valorization that reach everyone, because during the period they just lived many dramatic situations existed derived from the crisis, personal and family, that are attributed to the influence and prominence acquired by technology in the teaching-learning process; 6) the university regulatory framework will have to adapt to reality at all levels: governmental, autonomous and local; 7) it is necessary to be prepared, perfectly clear that the regulatory change to the *online* scenario will entail a profound system change, which will see how its architecture changes, with a structural configuration of the system appearing that will entail the definition of job, training and administrative profiles. and services (which may eventually lead to adjustments in the size of each university); 8) the transition to the *online* model requires investments; 9) the transition must be agreed with the other partners with which each university relate; 10) the change must incorporate interoperable technological solutions, coordinated at all levels of activity and in all sectors, that allow the different university communities of each university to interact, internal and externally.

116. New Zealand without COV: Five Steps to Avoid Taking Steps Back

Five keys to protecting long-term health follow [136]: 1) make public use of facemasks mandatory in certain situations; 2) improve the effectiveness of contact tracking with the right digital tools; 3) manage borders following a scientific approach; 4) create a national PH agency that be effective; 5) commit to deep transformation to avoid major global threats.

117. Strategic Value of Information in Epidemics Control in 20th Century

The public has the right to be informed in all truth, and the health professionals, the obligation to provide such information, and mainly to the public authorities, to make them understand the little vaccination efficacy to prevent or cut an outbreak, and that it is unnecessary in almost all of people's large populations; that what matters is solving the problem of public water supply of all their localities, which is profitable, and the fear of cholera outbreaks would be avoided and the endemic of their typhoid diseases would disappear [137]. An attitude of silence can only serve to disorient. In the press, the health situation must be discussed, applying optimistic accents if one wants, but as long as they do neither cause confusion nor hide the health practices in which they must participate more or less actively [138].

118. Why Do Women Resist COVID-19 Better? Answer May Lie on X Chromosome

Causes can be pointed to explain why men suffer more from COVID-19 [139]: 1) ACE2 may not be the only protein with receptor function for the virus; 2) ACE2 expression depends more on the absence of estradiol than on the number of X chromosomes; 3) postmenopausal women suffer less from the virus than men of the same age, yet their hormone levels are low; the explanation lies in the expression of its most numerous genes related to immune defense. Without ignoring other aspects, e.g., healthier lifestyle habits, hormones and a higher number of active genes linked to X chromosome provide women with greater protection and response capacity *vs.* this and other pathologies.

119. Collaboration across Disciplines Makes It Easier to Solve Problems

Interdisciplinary-work importance is so great that it becomes necessary to put it into practice from the moment of academic training [140]. Only in this way will people be able to tackle problems that present their origin in a single discipline, but their solution in the sum of the knowledge of several.

120. Learn to Care (of Each Other) in the New Time

The categorization of people's societies, in layers of greater or less vulnerability, puts them on alert and makes them think in common: people have no other choice [141]. Now more than ever, people were able to verify that what some suffer today, tomorrow they can suffer. Perhaps, for the first time and admitting that the reflection presents a selfish bias, people put themselves in the shoes of others because they saw the danger too close. Not bad. It is a wake up call to people's radically individualistic and materialistic societies. It is a siren of alarm from the sectors that demand people's attention because they cannot cope anymore. It is a call to take care (of each other), in addition to recognizing and applauding all efforts, to get out of people's own bubble and set their sights on those who suffer the most.

121. Three Topics on Technology That Should Be Reviewed

During COVID-19 pandemic, people saw clearly their dependence on technological development and discussed the hopes placed on techno-scientific advances. Topics that were repeated in recent times follow [142]: 1) technology is neither good nor bad, but everything depends on the use people make of it; 2) technology dehumanizes people (or, in another version, people must humanize technology); 3) technology already presents its own development dynamics, alien to any human control.

122. The Coronavirus Has Returned Women to the Domestic Sphere

The CoV returned women to the domestic sphere [143]. It is a wide crisis and can be long. A high risk exists that women lose much of what they achieved. People are rigid in their productive economy without the possibility of making hours flexible. In this section, domestic workers and caregivers are the most affected by poor wages. *The care is not resold and leaves no surplus value*. The stress is triple: 1) disease risk; 2) economic risk; 3) overcrowding.

123. COVID-19 Survey: Impact on Research Activity

M. Castelló, in EU Project *Researcher Identity Development*, designed a study to analyze how COVID-19 pandemic affected research activity in order to improve the support researchers receive. Questions follow. A. Impact of the COVID-19 pandemic on your emotional state (*cf.* Figure 17).

Q1. Since confinement began, have any of the following emotions intensified?

None Little Moderately Quite a lot Much

Restlessness or anguish

Sadness

Apathy or demotivation

Fatigue

Frustration

Helplessness, insecurity or hopelessness

Anger

Stress or burnout

Decayed executive functions (concentration, attention, memory, *etc.*)

Loneliness

To what extent do you think these emotions and sensations have affected your research activity?

Q2. In relation to your research activity, since the confinement began, have any of the following feelings changed?

It has decayed a lot

It has decayed

It has not had an impact

It has risen

It has risen a lot

Isolation or loneliness

Disconnection with research colleagues

Feeling of lack of guidance, accompaniment or supervision

Interest in my research/project(s)

Valuation/appreciation of my work

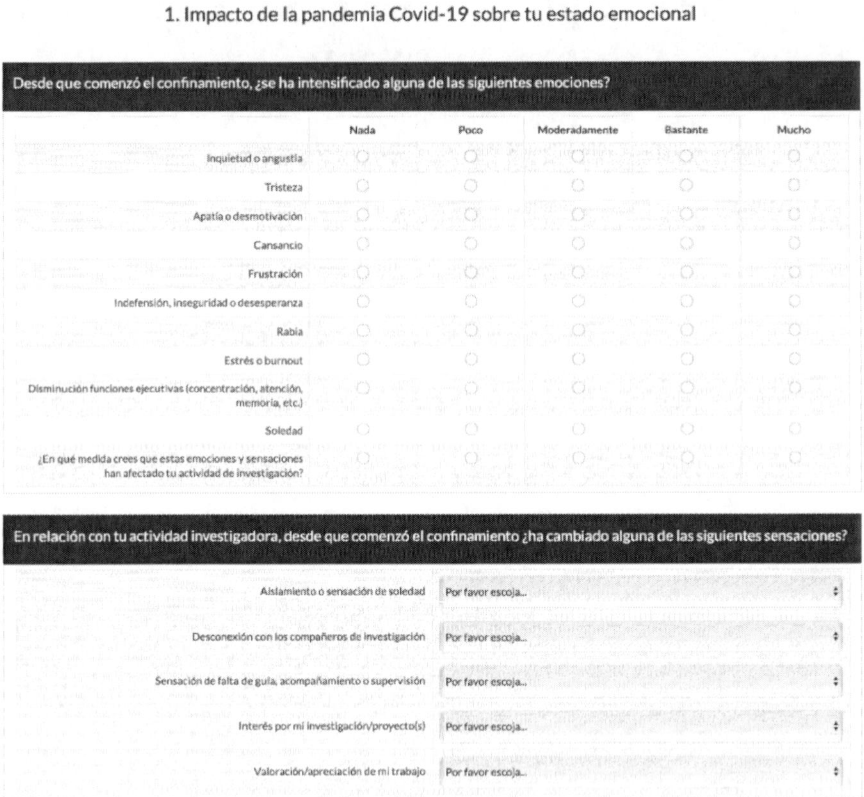

1. Impacto de la pandemia Covid-19 sobre tu estado emocional

Desde que comenzó el confinamiento, ¿se ha intensificado alguna de las siguientes emociones?

	Nada	Poco	Moderadamente	Bastante	Mucho
Inquietud o angustia	○	○	○	○	○
Tristeza	○	○	○	○	○
Apatía o desmotivación	○	○	○	○	○
Cansancio	○	○	○	○	○
Frustración	○	○	○	○	○
Indefensión, inseguridad o desesperanza	○	○	○	○	○
Rabia	○	○	○	○	○
Estrés o burnout	○	○	○	○	○
Disminución funciones ejecutivas (concentración, atención, memoria, etc.)	○	○	○	○	○
Soledad	○	○	○	○	○
¿En qué medida crees que estas emociones y sensaciones han afectado tu actividad de investigación?	○	○	○	○	○

En relación con tu actividad investigadora, desde que comenzó el confinamiento ¿ha cambiado alguna de las siguientes sensaciones?

Aislamiento o sensación de soledad	Por favor escoja...
Desconexión con los compañeros de investigación	Por favor escoja...
Sensación de falta de guía, acompañamiento o supervisión	Por favor escoja...
Interés por mi investigación/proyecto(s)	Por favor escoja...
Valoración/apreciación de mi trabajo	Por favor escoja...

Figure 17. Survey: Impact of the Covid-19 pandemic on your emotional state.

B. Impact of the Covid-19 pandemic on your research activity

Q3. What impact has Covid-19 pandemic had on the following aspects of your research activity?

Very negative impact
Negative impact
No impact
Positive impact
Very positive impact
Work rate
Deadlines
Planned activities and events
Reading scientific publications

Data collection or interventions

Data analysis

Productivity

Tasks of dissemination and communication of results

Preparation of applications for new projects or scholarships

Administrative tasks related to the adaptation of projects/scholarships that are underway

Labour or contractual conditions

Opportunities and future working conditions

Reconciliation of research with other professional tasks (e.g., teaching, tutoring, etc.)

Reconciliation of research with other tasks of personal or family life

Emergence of new topics related to the needs derived from the current situation

Prioritization of topics related to knowledge transfer

Interdisciplinary collaborations

Collaborations with researchers or other professionals from outside the academic field

Frequency of meetings

Efficiency of meetings

Q4. If there are others, please specify below (indicate them in the appropriate box according to their impact level):

It has had a very negative impact

It has had a negative impact

It has had a positive impact

It has had a very positive impact

Q5. Which of these changes do you think would be relevant if they were maintained? Why (indicate them in the appropriate box according to their impact level)?

Q6. What have you done to adjust to the changes you have indicated [name the (three) strategies that have served you best]?

Strategy 1

Strategy 2

Strategy 3

C. Supports

Q7. Regarding the following types of support, indicate if you have needed, received and/or sought them since the confinement began (you can mark as many columns as you think necessary).

Needed Received

Wanted None of the above

Economic and financial aid

Training materials and resources

Logistics help

Resources and technical assistance

Reconciliation of personal and work life

Emotional or personal

Q8. Have you received any other type of support? Please explain what support is involved and who has offered it to you.

D. Impact of the Covid-19 pandemic on research

Q9. Do you think Covid-19 had an impact on the research in your discipline in relation to the following aspects?

It has had a very negative impact

It has had a negative impact

It has not had an impact

It has had a positive impact

It has had a very positive impact

The appearance of new topics

The prioritization of knowledge transfer and dissemination

Interdisciplinary collaborations

Collaborations outside the academic field

Financing opportunities

Q10. If there are others, please specify below (indicate them in the appropriate box according to their impact level):

It has had a very negative impact
It has had a negative impact
It has had a positive impact
It has had a very positive impact

E. Impact of Covid-19 on the social perception of science and research

Q11. What impact do you think Covid-19 pandemic had on the interest in science and research of these groups?

It has had a very negative impact
It has had a negative impact
It has not had an impact
It has had a positive impact
It has had a very positive impact
Citizenship
Politicians
Media
Other professionals

Q12. Which of these changes do you think would be relevant if they were maintained? Why (indicate them in the appropriate box according to their impact level)?

124. People Must Use CoV Terrible Crisis to Rethink the Economic System

People must use COVID-19 terrible crisis as an opportunity to rethink the economic system [144]. It showed the high level of inequality that people present in their societies. People had to continue working or living on aid [145]. The extreme level of social inequalities imposes the need to change the economic system [146].

125. Why Children Avoid the Worst CoV Complications Might Lie in Arteries

Viral-elements presence in endothelial cells and an inflammatory-cells accumulation, with evidence of endothelial and inflammatory cell death, were shown, which suggests that SARS-CoV-2 infection facilitates endotheliitis induction in several organs as a direct consequence of viral involvement (noted with viral-bodies presence) and the host inflammatory response [147]. Apoptosis and pyroptosis induction might present an important role in endothelial cell injury in COVID-19 patients. Endotheliitis of COVID-19 could explain the systemic impaired microcirculatory function in different vascular beds and their clinical sequelae in COVID-19 patients, which hypothesis provides a rationale for therapies to stabilise the endothelium while tackling viral replication, particularly with anti-inflammatory anti-cytokine drugs, ACE inhibitors, and statins. The strategy could be particularly relevant for vulnerable patients with preexisting endothelial dysfunction, which is associated with male sex, smoking, hypertension, diabetes, obesity and established CVD, all associated with adverse outcomes in COVID-19. Evidence is mounting that healthy blood vessels protect children from serious COVID-19 effects, e.g., stroke [148].

126. Prevalence of Asymptomatic SARS-CoV-2 Infection: A Narrative Review

The SARS-CoV-2 spread rapidly throughout the world since the first COVID-19 cases were observed in Dec. 2019 in Wuhan, China. Infected persons who remain asymptomatic play a significant role in the ongoing pandemic, but their relative number and effect were uncertain. The available evidence on asymptomatic SARS-CoV-2 infection was reviewed and synthesized [149]. Asymptomatic persons seem to account for 40–45% of SARS-CoV-2 infections, and they can transmit the virus to others for an extended period, perhaps longer than 14d. Asymptomatic infection may be associated with subclinical lung abnormalities, as detected by computed tomography. Because of the high risk for silent spread by asymptomatic persons, it is imperative that testing programs include those without symptoms. To supplement conventional diagnostic testing, which is constrained by capacity, cost and its one-off nature, innovative tactics for PH surveillance (e.g., crowdsourcing digital wearable data, monitoring sewage sludge) might be helpful.

127. Keeping Governments Accountable: COVID-19 Assessment Scorecard

The COVID-19 response presents the potential to generate preparedness and response models for future PH emergencies, e.g., pandemics that are even more virulent [150]. The pandemic must be a wake-up call for countries to address the most critical shortcomings in their pandemic readiness and health-system resilience in order to prevent and mitigate the effects of future catastrophes.

128. Lessons from the Pandemic for EU: Risks of a Half-Baked Integration

Feás Costilla raised the following questions on the EU in the face of emergency and recovery [151].

Q1. What has been the EU's reaction to the emergency?

Q2. What should be the EU's strategy for recovery and what are the risks?

Q3. What does the CoV crisis teach us regarding the limitations of the EU integration process?

He provided the following conclusion (C):

C1. Crisis of CoV allowed people to see that EU in the face of an emergency is always capable of reacting, but it is unable to see threats that are just around the corner and propose ambitiously solutions that necessarily go *via* a higher level of integration.

129. Ideas for the Post-Pandemic: The Future That Awaits People

Lucena Giraldo and Martín-Aceña proposed hypotheses/questions/ answers on post-pandemic ideas [152].

H1. (Lucena Giraldo). History teaches people that they have experienced this before.

H2. (Lucena Giraldo). Globalization is not where people come from but where they are going.

H3. (Lucena Giraldo). The cultural is absolutely decisive.

H4. (Lucena Giraldo). The understanding of the pandemic is pulling the cultural.

H5. (Lucena Giraldo). *It is something they inflict on you!*

H6. (Lucena Giraldo). *It is not your fault!*

Q1. (Martín-Aceña). What is the future?

A1. (Martín-Aceña). The future is always uncertain.

H7. (Martín-Aceña). Globalization has spread the pandemic.

H8. (Martín-Aceña). Globalization is not going to back down.

H9. (Rodríguez LaFuente). Progress.

Q2. (Martín-Aceña). Is progress going to stop?

A2. (Martín-Aceña). No, people are facing a parenthesis as in the Black Death.

H10. (Rodríguez LaFuente). Virtual *vs.* face-to-face teaching.

H11. (Goethe). *I was there!*

H12. (Martín-Aceña). Virtuality is old, technology has only made it possible.

H13. (Lucena Giraldo). *Promised land* begins with confinement [Ellis Island, Hotel de Inmigrantes (Buenos Aires)].

H14. (Lucena Giraldo). People will survive if they have culture.

130. Does Density Aggravate COVID-19 Pandemic? Early Findings and Lessons

Density impact on emerging highly contagious infectious diseases was rarely studied. In theory, dense areas lead to more face-to-face interaction among residents, which makes them potential hotspots for the rapid pandemics spread. On the other hand, dense areas may present better access to HC facilities, and greater implementation of *social distancing* policies and practices. Pandemic of COVID-19 is a perfect case study to investigate the relationships. A study uses structural equation modelling to account for direct and indirect density impacts on COVID-19 infection, and mortality rates for 913 US metropolitan counties, controlling for key confounding factors [153]. Metropolitan population is one of the most significant predictors of infection rates; larger metropolitan areas present higher infection and mortality rates. After controlling for metropolitan population, county density is not significantly related to the infection rate, because of more adherence to *social distancing* guidelines. However, counties with higher densities present significantly lower virus-related mortality rates than do counties with lower densities, because of superior HC systems. Connectivity matters more than density in COVID-19-pandemic spread. Large metropolitan areas with a higher number of counties tightly linked together *via* economic, social and commuting relationships are the most vulnerable to the pandemic outbreaks. They are more likely to exchange tourists and businesspeople in themselves and with other parts, increasing the risk of cross-border infections. A key recommendation is that planners continue to advocate dense development for a host of reasons, e.g., lower death rates because of infectious diseases (COVID-19).

131. Immunoglobulin M/G-Antibodies Seroprevalence vs. SARS-CoV-2 in China

Detection of asymptomatic or subclinical SARS-CoV-2 infection is critical for understanding COVID-19 overall prevalence and infection potential. To estimate the cumulative prevalence of SARS-CoV-2 infection in China, the host serologic response was evaluated, measured by immunoglobulins M and G levels in 17 368 individuals, in the city of Wuhan, COVID-19-pandemic epicentre in China, and geographic regions in the country, in Mar. 9, 2020–Apr. 10, 2020 [154]. In the cohorts, the seropositivity in Wuhan varied in 3.2–3.8% in different subcohorts. Seroposivity progressively decayed in other cities as the distance to the epicentre rose. Patients who visited a hospital for maintenance hemodialysis and HC workers had a higher seroprevalence of 3.3 and 1.8%, respectively.

132. FDA-Approved Drug Ivermectin Inhibits SARS-CoV-2 Replication in Vitro

Although clinical trials are underway to test possible therapies, the worldwide response to COVID-19 outbreak was largely limited to monitoring/containment. Ivermectin, an FDA-approved anti-parasitic previously shown to present broad-spectrum anti-viral activity *in vitro*, is an inhibitor of the causative virus SARS-CoV-2, with a single addition to Vero-hSLAM cells 2h post-infection with SARS-CoV-2 able to effect 5000-fold reduction in viral RNA at 48h [155].

133. University: From Remote Emergency Teaching to Adapted Face-to-Face

The Association of University Informatics Teachers presented a statement that considers the following risks and opportunities for the next course [156]: 1) the rules must be flexible; 2) no need exists to overload teachers; 3) the focus should be on learning; 4) teacher education training needs to be increased; 5) social equity must be promoted.

134. That Disease Does Not Overcome Life: Lessons from History vs. Covid-19

A handful of lessons were drawn from history *vs.* COVID-1 [157]: 1) epidemics always existed; 2) one must be prepared (mentally, at least) for the worst; 3) how to act? 4) The consequences of the epidemic on people's lives must not be underestimated; 5) life goes on.

135. The Coronavirus Behaves Like a Sexually Transmitted Disease

Among all the mysteries surrounding COVID-19, one thing clear exists: People cannot let themselves be carried away by a false sense of security [158]. As Sun Tzu warns in *The Art of War*, one must know his enemy. People still must know a lot more about SARS-CoV-2 before they start to claim victory.

136. Modelling Infectious Epidemics

In a series of articles, Altman group discussed mathematical and statistical models that are commonly used to study the spread of infectious diseases [159]. Such models are used to inform decisions on disease prevention, surveillance, control and treatment, and can be applied to new epidemics, e.g., the ongoing COVID-19 outbreak.

137. Coronavirus Jolts Laboratories to Warp Speed

To thwart SARS-CoV-2, laboratories hurry to hone assays, swap findings and share resources [160]. Academic and industry laboratories are hurrying to address COVID-19 pandemic. The companies' culture are seen rising to the challenge of a pandemic. Extraction of RNA, among other tools and techniques, is important.

138. The Mind Matters

Mental health struggles represent a second pandemic in the wake of COVID-19 (people must stay connected as best they can, and extend a hand to those who need it) [161]. Pandemic of CoV repositioned health as public priority number one. Physical health, notwithstanding, represents only one part of the whole. In unprecedented *social-distancing* age, restricted movement and economic uncertainty, people must also take care to protect their mental health.

139. COVID-19: Improvise, Adapt and Overcome

Pandemic of COVID-19 brought with it drastic changes to all aspects of people's lives: How does this translate into their universities and conference programs? From the moment COVID-19 hit, scientists across disciplines were combining their expertise, racing to adapt to the evolving situation. The pandemic brought with it countless changes to people's personal and professional lives, but how are education and communication platforms adapting (and for how long will this be the case)? Robertson and van Geel heard from professors testing new technology to keep students informed and engaged, and explored how professors wrestled with dramatic changes to people's approach to conferences in 2020 [162].

140. Ruxolitinib for the Treatment of SARS-CoV-2-Induced ARDS

Artificial intelligence and pre-clinical studies suggested that baricitinib, a numb associated kinase and JAK1/2-inhibitor, inhibits clathrin-mediated endocytosis and antagonizes SARS-CoV-2 infection of cells. Besides ruxolitinib, baricitinib, which is approved in the treatment of rheumatoid arthritis, is another candidate with potential in COVID-19-disease treatment. However, since baricitinib may not penetrate into lung tissue, it was hypothesized that it may be less effective in COVID-19-associated ARDS [163]. The finding in a patient may present implications for the ongoing search for optimal therapy for patients suffering from severe COVID-19.

141. Robust T Cell Immunity in Individuals with Asymptomatic/Mild COVID-19

The SARS-CoV-2-specific memory T cells will likely prove critical for long-term immune protection *vs.* COVID-19. The functional and phenotypic landscape of SARS-CoV-2-specific T-cell responses were systematically mapped in a large cohort of unexposed individuals, and exposed family members and individuals with acute or convalescent COVID-19 [164]. Acute phase SARS-CoV-2-specific T cells displayed a highly activated cytotoxic phenotype, which correlated with a number of clinical markers of disease severity, whereas convalescent phase SARS-CoV-2-specific T cells were polyfunctional and displayed a stem-like memory phenotype. The SARS-CoV-2-specific T cells were detectable in antibody-seronegative family members, and individuals with an asymptomatic- or mild-COVID-19 history. The collective dataset shows that SARS-CoV-2 elicits robust memory T-cell responses akin to those observed in the context of successful vaccines, showing that natural exposure or infection may prevent recurrent severe-COVID-19 episodes also in seronegative individuals.

Conclusion

From the present results and discussion, the following final remarks can be drawn:

1) The presence of a large reservoir of severe acute respiratory syndrome-coronavirus-like viruses in horseshoe bats, and culture of eating exotic mammals in southern China, is a time bomb. The web dashboard is crucial to inform modelling efforts and control measures during the outbreak.
2) Globalization and climate change give rise to scenarios in which infectious agents present more opportunities to originate, and

facilitate spread of existing agents, which take the advantage to enhance their geographical spread and lead to worse pandemics. The changing world implies higher probabilities for such situations, and other epidemics or pandemics may appear in the future.

3) *Via* post-exposure hydroxychloroquine is in line with World Health Organisation's strategic objectives to limit human-to-human transmission. If people do not seriously consider using the easy and safe option, they are taking the risk of allowing the pandemic to sore out of control. The urgency of the epidemic necessitates choices about which interventions to employ.
4) Irrespective of the mechanisms by which severe acute respiratory syndrome-coronavirus-2 originated, the ongoing surveillance of pneumonia in humans and other animals is of importance.
5) Only experimental confirmation of the activity *in vitro* and *in vivo* of the compounds *vs.* the virus will demonstrate their real efficacy. However, the repositioning of drugs could shorten, significantly, the time in providing therapeutic alternatives to face the current public health crisis.
6) Awareness campaigns are created, hand hygiene products, supplied in public places in the form of gels and people, asked not to touch their faces with their hands. It must be understood that reducing every hundredth possible in the base presents a tremendous impact over time.
7) Zoonosis precautions: regulating live markets and guarding the animal borders of the viral world. Lowering the opportunity, people will stop the epidemic curve. Learning from history is essential even though they cannot prevent pathogens' natural evolution. These are the numbers that will save lives. Members of social nets share in the responsibility to address broader implications.

ACKNOWLEDGMENTS

The authors acknowledge Dr. Vicente Simón by the online courses *Mindfulness in Times of Crisis* and financial support from Fundación Universidad Católica de Valencia *San Vicente Mártir* (Project No. 2019-217-001UCV).

REFERENCES

[1] Arora, N.; Schuenemann, V. J.; Jäger, G.; Peltzer, A.; Seitz, A.; Herbig, A.; Strouhal, M.; Grillová, L.; Sánchez-Busó, L.; Kühnert, D.; Bos, K. I.; Rivero Davis, L.; Mikalová, L.; Bruisten, S.; Komericki, P.; French, P.; Grant, P. R.; Pando, M. A.; Gallo Vaulet, L.; Rodríguez Fermepin, M.; Martinez, A.; Centurion Lara, A.; Giacani, L.; Norris, S. J.; Smajs, D.; Bosshard, P. P.; González-Candelas, F.; Nieselt, K.; Krause, J.; Bagheri, H. C. Origin of modern syphilis and emergence of a pandemic *Treponema pallidum* cluster. *Nat. Microbiol.* 2017, 2, 16245–1-6.

[2] Patiño-Galindo J. Á.; Torres-Puente, M.; Bracho, M. A.; Alastrué, I.; Juan, A.; Navarro, D.; Galindo, M. J.; Ocete, D.; Ortega, E.; Gimeno, C.; Belda, J.; Domínguez, V.; Moreno, R.; González-Candelas, F. The molecular epidemiology of HIV-1 in the Comunidad Valenciana (Spain): Analysis of transmission clusters. *Sci. Rep.* 2017, 7, 11584–1-10.

[3] Patiño-Galindo, J. Á.; González-Candelas, F.; Pybus, O. G. The effect of RNA substitution models on viroid and RNA virus phylogenies. *Genome Biol. Evol.* 2018, 10, 657-666.

[4] Bassett, T. J.; Fogelman, C. Déjà vu or something new? The adaptation concept in the climate change literature. *Geoforum* 2013, 48, 42-53.

[5] Microscopy and Analysis. Coronavirus: How biologists resolved the virus so spectacularly quickly. *Microscop. Anal.* 2020, 2020(47), 18-20.

[6] Cheng, V. C. C.; Lau, S. K. P.; Woo, P. C. Y.; Yuen, K. Y. Severe acute respiratory syndrome coronavirus as an agent of emerging and reemerging infection. *Clin. Microbiol. Rev.* 2007, 20, 660-694.

[7] Johnson, C. K.; Hitchens, P. L.; Pandit, P. S.; Rushmore, J.; Evans, T. S.; Young, C. C. W.; Doyle, M. M. Global shifts in mammalian population trends reveal key predictors of virus spillover risk. *Proc. R. Soc. B* 2020, 287, 2736–1-10.

[8] Andersen, K. G.; Rambaut, A.; Lipkin, W. I.; Holmes, E. C.; Garry, R. F. The proximal origin of SARS-CoV-2. *Nat. Med.* 2020, 26, 450-452.

[9] Graham, R. L.; Baric, R. S. SARS-CoV-2: Combating coronavirus emergence. *Immunity*, in press.

[10] Dong, E.; Du, H.; Gardner, L. An interactive web-based dashboard to track COVID-19 in real time. *Lancet Infect. Dis.* 2020, 20, 533-534.

[11] Mas-Coma, S.; Jones, M. K.; Marty, A. M. COVID-19 and globalization. *One Health* 2020, 9, 100132–1-4.

[12] Picot, S.; Marty, A.; Bienvenu, A. L.; Blumberg, L. H.; Dupouy-Camet, J.; Carnevale, P.; Kano, S.; Jones, M. K.; Daniel-Ribeiro, C. T.; Mas-Coma, S. Coalition: Advocacy for prospective clinical trials to test the post-exposure potential of hydroxychloroquine against COVID-19. *One Health* 2020, 9, 100131–1-5.

[13] Galvez, J.; Zanni, R.; Galvez-Llompart, M. Drugs repurposing for coronavirus treatment: Computational study based on molecular topology. *Nereis* 2020, 2020(12), 15-18.

[14] Galisteo, A., personal communication.

[15] Kucharski, A. *The Rules of Contagion: Why Things Spread — and Why They Stop*; Profile: London, UK, 2020.

[16] Wenham, C. Modelling can only tell us so much: Politics explains the rest. *Lancet* 2020, 395, 1335-1335.

[17] Nay, O. Can a virus undermine human rights? *Lancet Public Health* 2020, 30092-X, 1-2.

[18] Graeden, E.; Carlson, C.; Katz, *R.* Answering the right questions for policymakers on COVID-19. *Lancet Glob. Health* 2020, 30191-1, 1-2.

[19] Limaye, R. J.; Sauer, M.; Ali, J.; Bernstein, J.; Wahl, B.; Barnhill, A.; Labrique, A. Building trust while influencing online COVID-19 content in the social media world. *Lancet Dig. Health* 2020, 30084–4, 1-2.

[20] Pareek, M.; Bangash, M. N.; Pareek, N.; Pan, D.; Sze, S.; Minhas, J. S.; Hanif, W.; Khunti, K. Ethnicity and COVID-19: An urgent public health research priority. *Lancet* 2020, 30922-3, 1-2.

[21] Wu, J. T.; Leung, K.; Leung, G. M. Nowcasting and forecasting the potential domestic and international spread of the 2019-nCoV outbreak originating in Wuhan, China: A modelling study. *Lancet* 2020, 395, 689-697.

[22] Horton. R. Offline: COVID-19 and the NHS—*A national scandal. Lancet* 2020, 395, 1022-1022.

[23] Zhang, Y. Z.; Koopmans, M.; Yuen, K. Y.; Andersen, K.; Perlman, S.; Hogue, B.; Eckerle, I. The novel coronavirus outbreak: What we know and what we don't. *Cell* 2020, 180, 1034-1036.

[24] The *Cell* Editorial Team. COVID-19: Navigating uncertainties together. *Cell* 2020, 181, 209-210.

[25] Callaghan, S. COVID-19 is a data science issue. *Patterns* 2020, 1, 100022–1-3.

[26] Liao, H.; Zhang, L.; Marley, G.; Tang, W. Differentiating COVID-19 response strategies. *Innovation*, in press.

[27] Oberfeld, B. Achanta, A.; Carpenter, K.; Chen, P.; Gilette, N.; Langat, P.; Said, J.; Schiff, A.; Zhou, A.; Barczak, A.; Pillai, S. COVID-19. *Cell*, in press.

[28] Blanco-Melo, D.; Nilsson-Payant, B. E.; Liu, W. C.; Uhl, S.; Hoagland, D.; Møller, R.; Jordan, T. X.; Oishi, K.; Panis, M.; Sachs, D.; Wang, T. T.; Schwartz, R. E.; Lim, J. K.; Albrecht, R. A.;

tenOever, B. R. Imbalanced host response to SARS-CoV-2 drives development of COVID-19. *Cell*, in press.

[29] Hoffmann, M.; Kleine-Weber, H.; Pöhlmann, S. A multibasic cleavage site in the spike protein of SARS-CoV-2 is essential for infection of human lung cells. *Mol. Cell*, in press.

[30] Ziegler, C. G. K.; Allon, S. J.; Nyquist, S. K.; Mbano, I. M.; Miao, V. N.; Tzouanas, C. N.; Cao, Y.; Yousif, A. S.; Bals, J.; Hauser, B. M.; Feldman, J.; Muus, C.; Wadsworth II, M. H.; Kazer, S. W.; Hughes, T. K.; Doran, B.; Gatter, G. J.; Vukovic, M.; Taliaferro, F.; Mead, B. E.; Guo, Z.; Wang, J. P.; Gras, D.; Plaisant, M.; Ansari, M.; Angelidis, I.; Adler, H.; Sucre, J. M. S.; Taylor, C. J.; Lin, B.; Waghray, A.; Mitsialis, V.; Dwyer, D. F.; Buchheit, K. M.; Boyce, J. A.; Barrett, N. A.; Laidlaw, T. M.; Carroll, S. L.; Colonna, L.; Tkachev, V.; Peterson, C. W.; Yu, A.; Zheng, H. B.; Gideon, H. P.; Winchell, C. G.; Lin, P. L.; Bingle, C. D.; Snapper, S. B.; Kropski, J. A.; Theis, F. J.; Schiller, H. B.; Zaragosi, L. E.; Barbry, P.; Leslie, A.; Kiem, H. P.; Flynn, J. L.; Fortune, S. M.; Berger, B.; Finberg, R. W.; Kean, L. S.; Garber, M.; Schmidt, A. G.; Lingwood, D.; Shalek, A. K.; Ordovas-Montanes, J.; HCA Lung Biological Network. SARS-CoV-2 receptor ACE2 is an interferon-stimulated gene in human airway epithelial cells and is detected in specific cell subsets across tissues. *Cell*, in press.

[31] Paraskevis, D.; Kostaki, E. G.; Magiorkinis, G.; Panayiotakopoulos, G.; Sourvinos, G.; Tsiodras, S. Full-genome evolutionary analysis of the novel corona virus (2019-nCoV) rejects the hypothesis of emergence as a result of a recent recombination event. *Infect. Genet. Evol.* 2020, 79, 104212–1-4.

[32] Chen, J. Pathogenicity and transmissibility of 2019-nCoV—A quick overview and comparison with other emerging viruses. *Microb. Infect*. 2020, 22, 69-71.

[33] Lai, C. C.; Shih, T. P.; Ko, W. C.; Tang, H. J.; Hsueh, P. R. Severe acute respiratory syndrome coronavirus 2 (SARS-CoV-2) and coronavirus disease-2019 (COVID-19): The epidemic and the challenges. *Int. J. Antimicrob. Agents* 2020, 55, 105924–1-9.

[34] Ashour, H. M.; Elkhatib, W. F.; Rahman, M.; Elshabrawy, H. A. Insights into the recent 2019 novel coronavirus (SARS-CoV-2) in light of past human coronavirus outbreaks. *Pathogens* 2020, 9, 186–1-15.

[35] Xie, M.; Chen, Q. Insight into 2019 novel coronavirus — An updated interim review and lessons from SARS-CoV and MERS-CoV. *Int. J. Infect. Dis*. 2020, 94, 119-124.

[36] Peckham, H.; de Gruijter, N. M.; Raine, C.; Radziszewska, A.; Ciurtin, C.; Wedderburn, L. R.; Rosser, E. C.; Deakin, C. T.; Webb, K. Sex-bias in COVID-19: A meta-analysis and review of sex differences in disease and immunity. *Lancet Infect. Dis*. submitted for publication.

[37] Li, Y.; Liu, B.; Cui, J.; Wang, Z.; Shen, Y.; Xu, Y.; Yao, K.; Guan, Y. COVID-19 evolves in human hosts, Xidian University–Peking University–University of Illinois at Chicago–University of Michigan, Working Paper, 2020, 1-24.

[38] Fuster, V.; Turco, J. V. COVID-19: A lesson in humility and an opportunity for sagacity and hope. *J. Am. Coll. Cardiol*., in press.

[39] Yong, C. COVID-19: The isolation that has brought us together. *J. Am. Coll. Cardiol*., in press.

[40] Thorlund, K.; Dron, L.; Park, J.; Hsu, G.; Forrest, J. I.; Mills, E. J. A real-time dashboard of clinical trials for COVID-19. *Lancet Dig. Health* 2020, 30086-8–1-2.

[41] Zhou, P.; Yang, X. L.; Wang, X. G.; Hu, B.; Zhang, L.; Zhang, W.; Si, H. R.; Zhu, Y.; Li, B.; Huang, C. L.; Chen, H. D.; Chen, J.; Luo, Y.; Guo, H.; Jiang, R. D.; Liu, M. Q.; Chen, Y.; Shen, X. R.; Wang, X.; Zheng, X. S.; Zhao, K.; Chen, Q. J.; Deng, F.; Liu, L. L.; Yan, B.; Zhan, F. X.; Wang, Y. Y.; Xiao, G. F.; Shi, Z. L. A pneumonia outbreak associated with a new coronavirus of probable bat origin. *Nature (London)* 2020, 579, 270-273.

[42] Hoffmann, M.; Kleine-Weber, H.; Schroeder, S.; Krüger, N.; Herrler, T.; Erichsen, S.; Schiergens, T. S.; Herrler, G.; Wu, N. H.; Nitsche, A.; Müller, M. A.; Drosten, C.; Pöhlmann, S. SARS-CoV-2

cell entry depends on ACE2 and TMPRSS2 and is blocked by a clinically proven protease inhibitor. *Cell* 2020, 181, 271-280.

[43] Hirano, T.; Masaaki Murakami, M. COVID-19: A new virus, but a familiar receptor and cytokine release syndrome. *Immunity*, in press.

[44] Sun, K.; Viboud, C. Impact of contact tracing on SARS-CoV-2 transmission. *Lancet Infect. Dis*. 2020, 30357-1.

[45] Altmann, D. M.; Douek, D. C.; Boyton, R. J. What policy makers need to know about COVID-19 protective immunity. *Lancet* 2020, 30985-5–1-3.

[46] Editorial. Isolation and inclusion. *Lancet Psychology* 2020, 7, 371-371.

[47] Townsend, E.; Nielsen, E.; Allister, R.; Cassidy, S. A. Key ethical questions for research during the COVID-19 pandemic. *Lancet Psychology* 2020, 7, 381-383.

[48] Markowitz, J. Virtual treatment and social distancing. *Lancet Psychology* 2020, 7, 388-389.

[49] Karamouzian, M.; Johnson, C.; Kerr, T. Public health messaging and harm reduction in the time of COVID-19. *Lancet Psychology* 2020, 7, 390-391.

[50] Editorial. Decolonising COVID-19. *Lancet Glob. Health* 2020, 8, e612–1-1.

[51] Netea, M. G.; Giamarellos-Bourboulis, E. J.; Domínguez-Andrés, J.; Curtis, N.; van Crevel, R.; van de Veerdonk, F. L.; Bonten, M. Trained immunity: A tool for reducing susceptibility and severity of SARS-CoV-2 infection. *Cell*, in press.

[52] Randolph, H. E.; Barreiro, L. B. Herd immunity: Understanding COVID-19. *Immunity*, in press.

[53] Huang, C.; Wang, Y.; Li, X.; Ren, L.; Zhao, J.; Hu, Y.; Zhang, L.; Fan, G.; Xu, J.; Gu, X.; Cheng, Z.; Yu, T.; Xia, J.; Wei, Y.; Wu, W.; Xie, X.; Yin, W.; Li, H.; Liu, M.; Xiao, Y.; Gao, H.; Guo, L.; Xie, J.; Wang, G.; Jiang, R.; Gao, Z.; Jin, Q.; Wang, J.; Cao, B. Clinical features of patients infected with 2019 novel coronavirus in Wuhan, China. *Lancet* 2020, 395, 497-506.

[54] Lu, R.; Zhao, X.; Li, J.; Niu, P.; Yang, B.; Wu, H.; Wang, W.; Song, H.; Huang, B.; Zhu, N.; Bi, Y.; Ma, X.; Zhan, F.; Wang, L.; Hu, T.; Zhou, H.; Hu, Z.; Zhou, W.; Zhao, L.; Chen, J.; Meng, Y.; Wang, J.; Lin, Y.; Yuan, J.; Xie, Z.; Ma, J.; Liu, W. J.; Wang, D.; Xu, W.; Holmes, E. C.; Gao, G. F.; Wu, G.; Chen, W.; Shi, W.; Tan, W. Genomic characterisation and epidemiology of 2019 novel coronavirus: Implications for virus origins and receptor binding. *Lancet* 2020, 395, 565-574.

[55] Basha, S. H. Molecular modeling and docking studies of DTQ, THQ, THY, TQ compounds compared with HCQ targeting receptor binding domain of SARS-CoV-2 drug target towards finding their potential to act as anti-coronavirus drug like small molecule, Report, Innovative Informatica Technologies: Hyderabad, India, 2020.

[56] Lvov, D. K.; Alkhovsky, S. V.; Kolobukhina, L. V.; Burtseva E. I. Etiology of epidemic outbreaks COVID-19 in Wuhan, Hubei province, Chinese People Republic associated with 2019-nCoV (*Nidovirales, Coronaviridae, Coronavirinae, Betacoronavirus*, subgenus *Sarbecovirus*): Lessons of SARS-CoV outbreak. *Voprosy Virusologii (Problems of Virology, Russian journal)* 2020, 65, 6-15.

[57] García Bello, D. No Tocar: *Ciencia contra la Desinformación en la Pandemia del* COVID-19; Paidós: Barcelona, Spain, 2020.

[58] WHO Working Group on Ethics and COVID-19. *Ethics and COVID-19: Resource allocation and priority-setting*, Tech. Rep. WHO/RFH/20.2, World Health Organization: Geneva, Switzerland, 2020.

[59] Fassin, D. *Life: A Critical User's Manual*; Wiley: Hoboken, NJ, 2018.

[60] Horton, R. Offline: A global health crisis? No, something far worse. *Lancet* 2020, 395, 1410-1410.

[61] Steffen, B.; Egli, F.; Pahle, M.; Schmidt, T. S. Navigating the clean energy transition in the COVID-19 crisis. *Joule* 2020, 4, 1-5.

[62] Chen, N.; Zhou, M.; Dong, X.; Qu, J.; Gong, F.; Han, Y.; Qiu, Y.; Wang, J.; Liu, Y.; Wei, Y.; Xia, J.; Yu, T.; Zhang, X.; Zhang, L. Epidemiological and clinical characteristics of 99 cases of 2019

novel coronavirus pneumonia in Wuhan, China: A descriptive study. *Lancet* 2020, 395, 507-513.

[63] Caly, L.; Druce, J.; Roberts, J.; Bond, K.; Tran, T.; Kostecki, R.; Yoga, Y.; Naughton, W.; Taiaroa, G.; Seemann, T.; Schultz, M. B.; Howden, B. P.; Korman, T. M.; Lewin, S. R.; Williamson, D. A.; Catton, M. G. Isolation and rapid sharing of the 2019 novel coronavirus (SARS-CoV-2) from the first patient diagnosed with COVID-19 in Australia. *Med. J. Aust.* 2020, 2-50569–1-4.

[64] Alemanno, A. The European response to COVID19: From regulatory emulation to regulatory coordination. *Eur. J. Risk Reg.* in press.

[65] Paules, C. I.; Marston, H. D.; Fauci, A. S. Coronavirus infections—More than just the common cold. *J. Am. Med. Assoc.* 2020, 323, 707-708.

[66] Pan, A.; Liu, L.; Wang, C.; Guo, H.; Hao, X.; Wang, Q.; Huang, J.; He, N.; Yu, H.; Lin, X.; Wei, S.; Wu, T. Association of public health interventions with the epidemiology of the COVID-19 outbreak in Wuhan, China. *J. Am. Med. Assoc.* 2020, 6130, E1-E9.

[67] Inglesby, T. V. Public health measures and the reproduction number of SARS-CoV-2. *J. Am. Med. Assoc.* 2020, 7878, E1-E2.

[68] Berwick, D. M. Choices for the *new normal*. *J. Am. Med. Assoc.* 2020, 6949, E1-E2.

[69] Editorial. COVID-19: Remaking the social contract. *Lancet* 2020, 395, 1401-1401.

[70] Editorial. COVID-19 puts societies to the test. *Lancet Public Health* 2020, 5, e235–1-1.

[71] Marston, C.; Renedo, A.; Miles, S. Community participation is crucial in a pandemic. *Lancet* 2020, 31054-0, 1-1.

[72] Ishiwatari, M.; Koike, T.; Hiroki, K.; Toda, T.; Katsube, T. Managing disasters amid COVID-19 pandemic: Approaches of response to flood disasters. *Prog. Disaster Sci.* 2020, 6, 100096–1-4.

[73] Ferretti, L.; Wymant, C.; Kendall, M.; Zhao, L.; Nurtay, A.; Abeler-Dörner, L.; Parker, M.; Bonsall, D.; Fraser, C. Quantifying SARS-

CoV-2 transmission suggests epidemic control with digital contact tracing. *Science* 2020, eabb6936–1-12.

[74] Xu, M.; Pirtskhalava, T.; Farr, J. N.; Weigand, B. M.; Palmer, A. K.; Weivoda, M. M.; Inman, C. L.; Ogrodnik, M. B.; Hachfeld, C. M.; Fraser, D. G.; Onken, J. L.; Johnson, K. O.; Verzosa, G. C.; Langhi, L. G. P.; Weigl, M.; Giorgadze, N.; LeBrasseur, N. K.; Miller, J. D.; Jurk, D.; Singh, R. J.; Allison, D. B.; Ejima, K.; Hubbard, G. B.; Ikeno, Y.; Cubro, H.; Garovic, V. D.; Hou, X.; Weroha, S. J.; Robbins, P. D.; Niedernhofer, L. J.; Khosla, S.; Tchkonia, T.; Kirkland, J. L. Senolytics improve physical function and increase lifespan in old age. *Nat. Med.* 2018, 24, 1246-1256.

[75] Verity, R.; Okell, L. C.; Dorigatti, I.; Winskill, P.; Whittaker, C.; Imai, N.; Cuomo-Dannenburg, G.; Thompson, H.; Walker, P. G. T.; Fu, H.; Dighe, A.; Griffin, J. T.; Baguelin, M.; Bhatia, S.; Boonyasiri, A.; Cori, A.; Cucunubá, Z.; FitzJohn, R.; Gaythorpe, K.; Green, W.; Hamlet, A.; Hinsley, W.; Laydon, D.; Nedjati-Gilani, G.; Riley, S.; van Elsland, S.; Volz, E.; Wang, H.; Wang, Y.; Xi, X.; Donnelly, C. A.; Ghani, A. C.; Ferguson, N. M. Estimates of the severity of coronavirus disease 2019: A model-based analysis. *Lancet Infect. Dis*. 2020, 30243-7–1-9.

[76] Mahase, E., Covid-19: Death rate is 0.66% and increases with age, study estimates. *Br. Med. J.* 2020, 369, m1327–1-1.

[77] Rabadan, R. *Understanding Coronavirus*; Cambridge University Press: Cambridge, UK, 2020.

[78] Bollyky, T. J.; Gostin, L. O.; Hamburg, M. A. The equitable distribution of COVID-19 therapeutics and vaccines. *J. Am. Med. Assoc*. 2020, 6641–E1-E2.

[79] Figueras Huerta, A.; Beatriz Novoa, B.; González Candelas, F. El virus de la COVID-19 ni se creó ni se escapó de un laboratorio. *Conversation* 2020, 2020(Apr. 20), 1-1. [The COVID-19 virus was neither created nor escaped from a laboratory.]

[80] Peretó, J. La COVID-19 i el costat fosc de la promiscuïtat de la vida. *Mètode* 2020, 1, 1-1. [COVID-19 and the dark side of the promiscuity of life.]

[81] Peretó, J. COVID-19 y el lado oscuro de la promiscuidad de la vida. *Conversation* 2020, 2020(May 20), 1-1. [COVID-19 and the dark side of life's promiscuity]

[82] Briones, C.; Peretó, J. El origen del coronavirus SARS-CoV-2, a la luz de la evolución. *Conversation* 2020, 2020(Apr. 21), 1-1. [The origin of the SARS-CoV-2 coronavirus, in light of evolution]

[83] Bosch, A.; Nieto, A.; Doménech Gómez, A. M.; Briones, C.; Alonso Martí, C.; Casas Flecha, I.; Buesa Gómez, J.; Navas Castillo, J.; López Guerrero, J. A.; Quer Sivila, J.; Echevarría Mayo, J. E.; Pallas Benet, V. Esto es lo que los virólogos sabemos hasta hoy sobre el coronavirus SARS-CoV-2. *Conversation* 2020, 2020(Apr. 28), 1-1. [This is what virologists know to date about the SARS-CoV-2 coronavirus.]

[84] Cabrera, M.; Poza, J. L.; Lloret, N. Docentes: Mutación o extinción. *Telos* 2020, 2020(112), 74-79. [Teachers: Mutation or extinction.]

[85] Cabrera, M.; Poza-Lujan, J. L.; Lloret Romero, N. Docentes universitarios en la era digital: Adaptarse o morir. *Conversation* 2020, 2020 (Jan. 9), 1-1. [University Teachers in the Digital Age: Adapt or Die.]

[86] Esteban Bara, F. COVID-19: La universidad debe renovarse en un entorno virtual sin perder su esencia. *Conversation* 2020, 2020(Apr. 28), 1-1. [COVID-19: The university must be renewed in a virtual environment without losing its essence]

[87] Beltrán, J., Venegas, M., Eds. Educar en época de confinamiento: La tarea de renovar un mundo común. *Revista de Sociología de la Educación-RASE* 2020, 13(2), 1-1. [Educating in times of confinement: The task of renewing a common world. *Journal of Sociology of Education-RASE*]

[88] Venegas, M.; Beltrán Llavador, J. Docentes, estudiantes y familias hablan sobre la educación no presencial. *Conversation* 2020, 2020(May 7), 1-1. [Teachers, students and families talk about non-face-to-face education.]

[89] Gonzalez Lopez-Valcarcel, B.; Tomaino, L.; Serra Majem, L.; Barber, P.; Rodríguez-Mireles, S. COVID-19: Pandemia de modelos matemáticos. *Conversation* 2020, 2020(Apr. 24), 1-1. [COVID-19: Mathematical modeling pandemic.]

[90] Rey Rocha, J.; Ladero, V.; Muñoz Ruiz, E. No todos los datos son iguales: La importancia del contexto en la información sobre la pandemia. *Conversation* 2020, 2020(May 7), 1-1. [Not all facts are the same: The importance of context in information about the pandemic.]

[91] An, J.; Liao, X.; Xiao, T.; Qian, S.; Yuan, J.; Ye, H.; Qi, F.; Shen, C.; Liu, Y.; Wang, L.; Cheng, X.; Li, N.; Cai, Q.; Wang, F.; Chen, J.; Liu, Y.; Wang, Y.; Zhang, F.; Fu, Y.; Tan, X.; Liu, L.; Zhang, Z. Clinical characteristics of the recovered COVID-19 patients with re-detectable positive RNA test. *medRxiv* 2020, 2020, 2020.03.26. 20044222–1-29.

[92] Ministerio de Sanidad. *Buenas Prácticas en los Centros de Trabajo: Medidas para la Prevención de Contagios del COVID-19*, Guía No. 1104, Ministerio de Sanidad: Madrid, Spain, 2020. [*Good Practices in the Workplace: Measures for the Prevention of Contagions of COVID-19*]

[93] Ministerio de Sanidad. *Procedimiento de Actuación para los Servicios de Prevención de Riesgos Laborales frente a la Exposición al SARS-CoV-2*; Ministerio de Sanidad: Madrid, Spain, 2020. [*Action Procedure for Occupational Risk Prevention Services against Exposure to SARS-CoV-2*]

[94] Moreno Tarín, S. L'arribada de la COVID-19 en un context d'emergència climàtica: Les conseqüències d'una crisi de crisis. *Mètode* 2020, 1, 1-1. [The arrival of COVID-19 in a context of climate emergency: The consequences of a crisis crisis.]

[95] WHO. *Gender and COVID-19: Advocacy brief*, Tech. Rep. WHO/2019-nCoV/Advocacy_brief/Gender/2020.1, World Health Organization: Geneva, Switzerland, 2020.

[96] Ledford, H. Autopsy slowdown hinders quest to determine how coronavirus kills. *Nature (London)* 2020, 2020, d41586-020-01355-z–1-1.

[97] Xie, P.; Ma, W.; Tang, H.; Liu, D. Severe COVID-19: A review of recent progress with a look toward the future. *Front. Public Health* 2020, 8, 189–1-7.

[98] Saad-Roy, C. M.; Wingreen, N. S.; Levin, S. A.; Grenfell, B. T. Dynamics in a simple evolutionary-epidemiological model for the evolution of an initial asymptomatic infection stage. *Proc. Natl. Acad. Sci. U.S.A.* 2020, 2020, 1920761117–1-1.

[99] Stadnytskyi, V.; Bax, C. E.; Bax, A.; Anfinrud, P. The airborne lifetime of small speech droplets and their potential importance in SARS-CoV-2 transmission. *Proc. Natl. Acad. Sci. U.S.A.* 2020, 2020, 2006874117–1-3.

[100] Zhou, H.; Chen, X.; Hu, T.; Li, J.; Song, H.; Liu, Y.; Wang, P.; Liu, D.; Yang, J.; Holmes, E. C.; Hughes, A. C.; Bi, Y.; Shi, W. A novel bat coronavirus closely related to SARS-CoV-2 contains natural insertions at the S1/S2 cleavage site of the spike protein. *Curr. Biol.* 2020, 30, 1-8.

[101] Liu, P.; Jiang, J. Z.; Wan, X. F.; Hua, Y.; Li, L.; Zhou, J.; Wang, X.; Hou, F.; Chen, J.; Zou, J.; Chen, J. Are pangolins the intermediate host of the 2019 novel coronavirus (SARS-CoV-2)? *PLoS Pathog.* 2020, 16, e1008421–1-13.

[102] Pinto, D. Park, Y. J.; Beltramello, M.; Walls, A. C.; Tortorici, M. A.; Bianchi, S.; Jaconi, S.; Culap, K.; Zatta, F.; De Marco, A.; Peter, A.; Guarino, B.; Spreafico, R.; Cameroni, E.; Case, J. B.; Chen, R. E.; Havenar-Daughton, C.; Snell, G.; Telenti, A.; Virgin, H. W.; Lanzavecchia, A.; Diamond, M. S.; Fink, K.; Veesler, D.; Corti, D. Cross-neutralization of SARS-CoV-2 by a human monoclonal SARS-CoV antibody. *Nature (London)*, in press.

[103] Máñez, E.; Lorenzo, M.; Ariño, A., personal communication.

[104] Barona, J. L. Lliçons de la pandemia. *eldiario.es* 2020, 2020(Apr. 11), 1-1. [Lessons from the pandemic]

[105] Chiumello, D.; Carlesso, E.; Brioni, M.; Cressoni, M. Airway driving pressure and lung stress in ARDS patients. *Critical Care* 2016, 20, 276–1-10.

[106] Amato, M. B. P.; Meade, M. O.; Slutsky, A. S.; Brochard, L.; Costa, E. L. V.; Schoenfeld, D. A.; Stewart, T. E.; Briel, M.; Talmor, D.; Mercat, A.; Richard, J. C. M.; Carvalho, C. R. R.; Brower, R. G. Driving pressure and survival in the acute respiratory distress syndrome. *N. Engl. J. Med.* 2015, 372, 747-755.

[107] Seheult, J.; Fitzpatrick, G.; Boran, G. Lactic acidosis: An update. *Clin. Chem. Lab. Med.* 2017, 55, 322-333.

[108] Combes, A.; Hajage, D.; Capellier, G.; Demoule, A.; Lavoué, S.; Guervilly, C.; Da Silva, D.; Zafrani, L.; Tirot, P.; Veber, B.; Maury, E.; Levy, B.; Cohen, Y.; Richard, C.; Kalfon, P.; Bouadma, L.; Mehdaoui, H.; Beduneau, G.; Lebreton, G.; Brochard, L.; Ferguson, N. D.; Fan, E.; Slutsky, A. S.; Brodie, D.; Mercat, A. for the EOLIA Trial Group, REVA, ECMONet. Extracorporeal membrane oxygenation for severe acute respiratory distress syndrome. *N. Engl. J. Med.* 2018, 378, 1965-1975.

[109] García, F. E.; Cova, F.; Rincón, P.; Vázquez, C. Trauma or growth after a natural disaster? The mediating role of rumination processes. *Eur. J. Psychotraum.* 2015, 6, 26557–1-10.

[110] Vázquez, C. ¿Trauma o crecimiento personal? Futuros posibles tras una pandemia. *Conversation* 2020, 2020(Apr. 22), 1-1. [Trauma or personal growth? Possible futures after a pandemic.]

[111] Laparra Navarro, M. ¿Qué transformaciones sociales nos traerá esta crisis del coronavirus? *Traductor de Ciencia* 2020, 2020(Mar. 31), 1-1. [What social transformations will this coronavirus crisis bring us?]

[112] Laparra Navarro, M. ¿Qué transformaciones sociales nos traerá el coronavirus? *Conversation* 2020, 2020(Apr. 22), 1-1. [What social transformations will the coronavirus bring us?]

[113] Sasia, P. M.; Bilbao Alberdi, G. Educación *online* frente a presencial: No hay lugar como la escuela para aprender.

Conversation 2020, 2020(Apr. 27), 1-1. [Online versus face-to-face education: There is no place like school to learn.]

[114] Moreno Pestaña J. L.; de Pinedo García, M.; Villanueva Fernández, N. ¿Quién teme al bulo feroz? *Conversation* 2020, 2020(Apr. 27), 1-1. [Who's afraid of the ferocious hoax?]

[115] Mehra, M. R.; Desai, S. S.; Kuy, S.; Henry, T. D.; Patel, A. N. Cardiovascular disease, drug therapy, and mortality in Covid-19. *N. Engl. J. Med.* 2020, 2007621–1-8.

[116] Mehra, M. R.; Desai, S. S.; Ruschitzka, F.; Patel, A. N. Hydroxychloroquine or chloroquine with or without a macrolide for treatment of COVID-19: A multinational registry analysis. *Lancet* 2020, 31180-6–1-10.

[117] Aleta, A.; Martín-Corral, D.; Pastore y Piontti, A.; Ajelli, M.; Litvinova, M.; Chinazzi, M.; Dean, N. E.; Halloran, M. E.; Longini, I. M., Jr.; Merler, S.; Pentland, A.; Vespignani, A.; Moro, E.; Moreno, Y. Modeling the impact of social distancing, testing, contact tracing and household quarantine on second-wave scenarios of the COVID-19 epidemic. *medRxiv* 2020, 2020(05.06), 20092841–1-31.

[118] Amat, F.; Arenas, A.; Falcó-Gimeno, A.; Muñoz, J. Pandemics meet democracy: Experimental evidence from the COVID-19 crisis in Spain. *SocArXiv* 2020, 2020(0504), dkusw–1-31.

[119] Van Leeuwen, F.; Petersen, M. B. The behavioral immune system is designed to avoid infected individuals, not outgroups. *Evol. Hum. Behav.* 2018, 39, 226-234.

[120] Grifoni, A.; Weiskopf, D.; Ramirez, S. I.; Mateus, J.; Dan, J. M.; Moderbacher, C. R.; Rawlings, S. A.; Sutherland, A.; Premkumar, L.; Jadi, R. S.; Marrama, D.; de Silva, A. M.; Frazier, A.; Carlin, A.; Greenbaum, J. A.; Peters, B.; Krammer, F.; Smith, D. M.; Crotty, S.; Sette, A. Targets of T cell responses to SARS-CoV-2 coronavirus in humans with COVID-19 disease and unexposed individuals. *Cell*, in press.

[121] Chandrashekar, A.; Liu, J.; Martinot, A. J.; McMahan, K.; Mercado, N. B.; Peter, L.; Tostanoski, L. H.; Yu, J.; Maliga, Z.; Nekorchuk,

M.; Busman-Sahay, K.; Terry, M.; Wrijil, L. M.; Ducat, S.; Martinez, D. R.; Atyeo, C.; Fischinger, S.; Burke, J. S.; Slein, M. D.; Pessaint, L.; Van Ry, A.; Greenhouse, J.; Taylor, T.; Blade, K.; Cook, A.; Finneyfrock, B.; Brown, R.; Teow, E.; Velasco, J.; Zahn, R.; Wegmann, F.; Abbink, P.: Bondzie, E. A.; Dagotto, G.; Gebre, M. S.; He, X.; Jacob-Dolan, C.; Kordana, N.; Li, Z.; Lifton, M. A.; Mahrokhian, S. H.; Maxfield, L. F.; Nityanandam, R.; Nkolola, J. P., Schmidt, A. G.; Miller, A. D.; Baric, R. S.; Alter, G.; Sorger, P. K.; Estes, J. D., Andersen, H., Lewis, M. G.; Barouch, D. H. SARS-CoV-2 infection protects against rechallenge in rhesus macaques. *Science* 2020, 2020, abc4776–1-11.

[122] García, M. J., personal communication.

[123] Wrapp, D. Wang, N.; Corbett, K. S.; Goldsmith, J. A.; Hsieh, C. L.; Abiona, O.; Graham, B. S.; McLellan, J. S. Cryo-EM structure of the 2019-nCoV spike in the prefusion conformation. *Science* 2020, 367, 1260-1263.

[124] Walls, A. C.; Park, Y. J.; Tortorici, M. A.; Wall, A.; McGuire, A. T.; Veesler, D. Structure, function, and antigenicity of the SARS-CoV-2 spike glycoprotein. *Cell* 2020, 181, 281-292.

[125] Hsiang, S.; Allen, D.; Annan-Phan, S.; Bell, K.; Bolliger, I.; Chong, T.; Druckenmiller, H.; Huang, L. Y.; Hultgren, A.; Krasovich, E.; Lau, P.; Lee, J.; Rolf, E.; Tseng; J.; Wu, T. The effect of large-scale anti-contagion policies on the COVID-19 pandemic. *Nature (London)* 2020_s41586-020-2404-8–1-8.

[126] Soriano, V. ¿Es COVID-19 cada vez más benigna? *Conversation* 2020, 2020(Jun. 10), 1-1. [Is COVID-19 getting more benign?]

[127] Ministerio de Trabajo y Economía Social. *Consulta pública previa a la elaboración de un proyecto normativo consistente en la modificación y elaboración de las condiciones para prestar trabajo por cuenta ajena a distancia*, Ministerio de Trabajo y Economía Social, Madrid, Spain, 2020. [Ministry of Labor and Social Economy. *Public consultation prior to the preparation of a normative project consisting of the modification and elaboration of*

the conditions to provide work for others at a distance, Ministry of Labor and Social Economy]

[128] De Sousa Santos, B. *La Cruel Pedagogía del Virus*; CLACSO: Buenos Aires, Argentina, 2020. [*The Cruel Pedagogy of the Virus*]

[129] Nsoesie, E. O.; Rader, B.; Barnoon, Y. L. Goodwin, L.; Brownstein, J. S. *Analysis of hospital traffic and search engine data in Wuhan China indicates early disease activity in the Fall of 2019*, Inst. Repos. 42669767, Harvard University: Cambridge, MA, 2020.

[130] Arsuaga, J. L.; Martinón-Torres, M. Homeostasis y crisis del coronavirus. *Conversation* 2020, 2020(Apr. 28), 1-1. [Homeostasis and the coronavirus crisis]

[131] Claret, J. La historia de la Humanidad es una sucesión de pandemias, pero no aprendemos. *Conversation* 2020, 2020(May 7), 1-1. [The history of Humanity is a succession of pandemics, but we do not learn]

[132] Aramayo, R. R. COVID-19 nos recuerda que no somos dioses (y es una buena noticia). *Conversation* 2020, 2020(May 10), 1-1. [COVID-19 reminds us that we are not gods (and it is good news).]

[133] Caireta Serra, S.; Font, M. La bioinformática se une a la lucha contra la COVID-19. *Conversation* 2020, 2020(Jun. 6), 1-1. [Bioinformatics joins the fight against COVID-19]

[134] Comas Espadas, I.; Chiner Oms, Á.; García Marín, A. M.; González Candelas, F. ¿Qué sabemos hasta hoy sobre la transmisión del SARS-CoV-2? *Conversation* 2020, 2020(Jun. 7), 1-1. [What do we know to date about the transmission of SARS-CoV-2?]

[135] Verdegay Galdeano, J. L. Diez ideas para un tránsito digital exitoso de las universidades. *Conversation* 2020, 2020(Jun. 8), 1-1. [Ten ideas for a successful digital transit of universities.]

[136] Baker, M.; Wilson, N. Nueva Zelanda sin coronavirus: Cinco medidas para no dar pasos atrás. *Conversation* 2020, 2020(Jun. 8), 1-1. [New Zealand without coronavirus: Five steps not to take steps back.]

[137] Heredia Flores, V. M. El valor estratégico de la información en el control de las epidemias del siglo XX. *Conversation* 2020,

2020(Jun. 8), 1-1. [The strategic value of information in the control of the epidemics of the 20th century.]

[138] Heredia Flores, V. M. El valor estratégico de la información en el control de las epidemias del siglo XX. *La Verdad* 2020, 2020(Jun. 9), 1-1. [The strategic value of information in the control of the epidemics of the 20th century.]

[139] Uranga, J. A. ¿Por qué las mujeres resisten mejor la COVID-19? La respuesta puede estar en el cromosoma X. *Conversation* 2020, 2020(Jun. 9), 1-1. [Why are women better resistant to COVID-19? The answer may lie on the X chromosome.]

[140] Arribillaga, A.; Aizpurua Sanz, A.; Aróstegui Barandica, I.; Jaureguizar Alboniga-Mayor, J.; Guerra Bilbao, N.; Berasategui Sancho, N. La colaboración entre disciplinas facilita resolver problemas (incluso la COVID-19). *Conversation* 2020, 2020(Jun. 10), 1-1. [Collaboration between disciplines makes it easy to solve problems (including COVID-19).]

[141] Pagola Carte, J. I. Aprender a cuidar(nos) en el nuevo tiempo. *Conversation* 2020, 2020(Jun. 10), 1-1. [Learn to care for (ourselves) in the new time.]

[142] Diéguez Lucena, A. Tres tópicos sobre la tecnología que conviene revisar. *Conversation* 2020, 2020(Jun. 10), 1-1. [Three topics about technology that should be reviewed.]

[143] Durán, Á., personal communication.

[144] Piketty, T., personal communication.

[145] Piketty, T., *Le Capital au XXIe Siècle*; Éditions du Seuil: Paris, France, 2013. [*Capital in the 21st Century*]

[146] Piketty, T., *Capital e Ideología*; Ediciones Deusto: Barcelona, Spain, 2019. [*Capital and Ideology*]

[147] Varga, Z.; Flammer, A. J.; Steiger, P.; Haberecker, M.; Andermatt, R.; Zinkernagel, A. S.; Mehra, M. R.; Schuepbach, R. A.; Ruschitzka, F.; Moch, H. Endothelial cell infection and endotheliitis in COVID-19. *Lancet* 2020, 395, 1417-1418.

[148] Cyranoski, D. Why children avoid the worst coronavirus complications might lie in their arteries. *Nat. Res.* 2020, d41586-020-01692-z–1-1.

[149] Oran, D. P.; Topol, E. J. Prevalence of asymptomatic SARS-CoV-2 infection: A narrative review. *Ann. Intern. Med.* 2020, M20-3012–1-1.

[150] Lazarus, J. V.; Binagwaho, A.; El-Mohandes, A. A. E.; Fielding, J. E.; Larson, H. J.; Plasència, A.; Andriukaitis, V.; Ratzan. S. C. Keeping governments accountable: The COVID-19 Assessment Scorecard (COVID-SCORE). *Nat. Med.* 2020, s41591-020-0950-0–1-4.

[151] Feás Costilla, E., personal communication.

[152] Lucena Giraldo, M.; Martín-Aceña, P., personal communication.

[153] Hamidi, S.; Sabouri, S.; Ewing, R. Does density aggravate the COVID-19 Pandemic? Early findings and lessons for planners. *J. Am. Plan. Assoc.* 2020, 1777891–1-15.

[154] Xu, X.; Sun, J.; Nie, S.; Li, H.; Kong, Y.; Liang, M.; Hou, J.; Huang, X.; Li, D.; Ma, T.; Peng, J.; Gao, S.; Shao, Y.; Zhu, H.; Lau, J. Y. N.; Wang, G.; Xie, C.; Jiang, L.; Huang, A.; Yang, Z.; Zhang, K.; Hou, F. F. Seroprevalence of immunoglobulin M and G antibodies against SARS-CoV-2 in China. *Nat. Med.* 2020, s41591-020-0949-6.

[155] Caly, L.; Druce, J. D.; Catton, M. G.; Jans, D. A.; Wagstaff, K. M. The FDA-approved drug ivermectin inhibits the replication of SARS-CoV-2 *in vitro*. *Antiv. Res.* 2020, 178, 104787–1-4.

[156] Sánchez Carracedo, F.; López Álvarez, D.; Llorens Largo, F.; Badía Contelles; J. M.; Marco Galindo, M. J. La universidad que viene: De la *docencia remota de emergencia* a la *presencialidad adaptada*. *Conversation* 2020, 2020(Jun. 18), 1-1. [The University to Come: From Emergency Remote Teaching to Adapted Presence.]

[157] López Zapico, M. A.; Hernández, M. Que la enfermedad no venza a la vida: Cinco lecciones de la Historia frente a la COVID-19. *Conversation* 2020, 2020(Jun. 22), 1-1. [That the disease does not defeat life: Five lessons from History against COVID-19.]

[158] Aktipis, A.; Alcock, J. El coronavirus se comporta como una enfermedad de transmisión sexual. *Conversation* 2020, 2020(Jun. 23), 1-1. [The coronavirus behaves like a sexually transmitted disease]

[159] Bjørnstad, O. N.; Shea, K.; Krzywinski, M.; Altman, N. Modeling infectious epidemics. *Nature Meth.* 2020, 17, 455-456.

[160] Marx, V. Coronavirus jolts labs to warp speed. *Nature Meth.* 2020, 17, 465-468.

[161] Hallam, M. The mind matters. *Anal. Scientist* 2020, 2020(87), 3-3.

[162] Robertson, L.; van Geel, F. COVID-19: Improvise, adapt, overcome. *Anal. Scientist* 2020, 2020(87), 14-23.

[163] Neubauer, A.; Wiesmann, T.; Vogelmeier, C. F.; Mack, E.; Skevaki, C.; Gaik, C.; Keller, C.; Figiel, J.; Sohlbach, K.; Rolfes, C.; Renz, H.; Wulf, H.; Burchert, A. Ruxolitinib for the treatment of SARS-CoV-2 induced acute respiratory distress syndrome (ARDS). *Leukemia* 2020, s41375-020-0907-9–1-3.

[164] Sekine, T.; Perez-Potti, A.; Rivera-Ballesteros, O.; Strålin, K.; Gorin, J. B.; Olsson, A.; Llewellyn-Lacey, S.; Kamal, H.; Bogdanovic, G.; Muschiol, S.; Wullimann, D. J.; Kammann, T.; Emgård, J.; Parrot, T.; Folkesson, E.; Rooyackers, O.; Eriksson, L. I.; Sönnerborg, A.; Allander, T.; Albert, J.; Nielsen, M.; Klingström, J.; Gredmark-Russ, S.; Björkström, N. K.; Sandberg, J. K.; Price, D. A.; Ljunggren, H. G.; Aleman, S.; Buggert, M.; Karolinska COVID-19 Study Group. Robust T cell immunity in convalescent individuals with asymptomatic or mild COVID-19. *bioRxiv* 2020, 06.29.174888–1-3.

In: COVID-19 Pandemic
Editor: A. K. Haghi

ISBN: 978-1-53618-565-2

Chapter 2

Influence of Allopathy, Homeopathy, Ayurveda and Unani Systems of Medicine in the Management of COVID-19

Eknath D. Ahire[1,*], Khemchand R. Surana[2], Vijayraj N. Sonawane[2], Khushali R. Pagar[1], Sachin S. Gunjal[1] and Swati G. Talele[3]

[1*]Department of Pharmaceutics, SSS's, Divine College of Pharmacy, Satana, India

[2]Department of Phamaceutical Chemistry, SSS's, Divine College of Pharmacy, Satana, India

[3]Department of Pharmaceutics, Sandip Institute of Pharmaceutical Sciences, Nashik, Maharashtra, India

---

[*] Corresponding Author's E-mail: eknathahire05@gmail.com.

ABSTRACT

COVID-19 is a viral disease occurring due to Severe Acute Respiratory Syndrome Coronavirus 2 virus. The patients founds with flu-like symptoms with a high fever, dry cough, painful throat, and breathing related difficulties. It caused by SARS-CoV-2 was known as COVID-19. Even though countless efforts, till there is no specialized treatment for COVID-19. Though, prevention and management are the only options as of now. This Chapter describes SARS-CoV-2, prevention and management treatment by using different medical systems like Allopathy, Ayurveda, Homeopathy and Unani. It was well reported that a combination of antiviral drugs along with hydroxyl-chloroquine and azithromycin by the proper consultation of a medical practitioner, may be the choice to treat the patients, as per the patient's situations and indications. Nevertheless, Unani treatment may be also beneficial with allopathic treatment. It is straightaway directed and demanded by different government bodies that all the persons should obey the preventive measures, managements rigorously without any discrepancy else the condition may be the worst. Correspondingly, there is an urgent requirement to find more novel and innovative treatment by using Allopathy, Ayurveda, Homeopathy and Unani medicine systems. Because there urgent need develops proper prevention and management strategies to combat this pandemic. This clause may be worthwhile to get awareness about prevention, manage and treatment of COVID-19.

Keywords: COVID-19, Ayurveda, Unani, homeopathy, Allopathy, treatment

ABBREVIATIONS

ARDS	Acute Respiratory Distress Syndrome
COVID-19	Coronavirus 2
FDA	Food and Drug Administration
ICU	Intensive Care Unit
IFN	Interferon
IMV	Invasive Mechanical Ventilation
MERS	Middle East Respiratory Syndrome
NIH	National Institutes of Health

NIV	Noninvasive
RCT	Randomized Controlled Treatment
RSV	Respiratory Syncytial Virus
SARS	Severe Acute Respiratory Syndrome
SARS-CoV-2	Severe Acute Respiratory Syndrome Coronavirus 2
UV	Ultraviolet

1. Background

The prevention and management are most significant concerns to control COVID-19. So, in that location is an abundant requirement for the co-operative efforts of the medical professionals and scientists with the regimen. The right medicines are actually essential to keep in this tragedy. In that location is no precise treatment suggested for COVID-19, and no vaccine is presently available. The treatment is symptomatic, and oxygen therapy signifies the beginning step in managing respiratory deficiency. Noninvasive (NIV) and invasive mechanical ventilation (IMV) may be essential in cases of respiratory failure refractory to oxygen treatment. Once more, intensive care is desirable to deal with complex forms of the disease [1, 2].

Regarding acute respiratory distress syndrome (ARDS) treatment, collecting knowledge on the pathophysiology of lung deterioration, have progressively induced clinicians to review approaches for working with respiratory failure. This characteristic of the disease is of major significance and has possibly negatively exaggerated the therapeutic methodology in the initial stages of the pandemic. Definitely, despite at commencement of the pandemic, primary IMV was assumed as the best approach for addressing CARDS, in COVID-19 pneumonia the characteristic ARDS respiratory mechanics showing abridged lung compliance (i.e., Capability to extend and enlarge lungs) can't be installed. On the conflicting, in CARDS, worthy pulmonary amenability can be reached. As a significance, and in dissimilarity to what was primarily supposed, NIV can have a key role in CARDS therapy [3].

At present, treatment delivered to the exaggerated individuals are primarily symptom grounded, and the extremely ill persons are providing with organ support [4]. It is essential to devote time and effort in finding vaccines and drugs for this novel virus. Meanwhile the development of drugs precise for COVID -19 will take more few months, drugs which have been established to be safe for humans can be repurposed to treat this disease. The enormous majority of the drugs applied for treatment wide-reaching falls under any of the bellow classification of drugs [5]. More research may be essential in existing medicine to apply them in the treatment of COVID-19 [6].

This Chapter recaps existing indication regarding major proposed different treatments, repurposed drugs for COVID-19 and offers a summary of current treatment management for this novel pandemic coronavirus.

2. Treatment Objectives

In that situation is no exact treatment for coronavirus, but prevention, management and supporting health care may provide ease in the outbreak of COVID-19. All the same, some approaches have been or may be used to control this disease. These attacks may be categorized in Allopathic, Unani and Homeopathic treatments. But before all this treatment, plenty of testing facilities should be available to the health care sectors [1].

3. Allopathic Treatment

Allopathic treatment and management comprise oxygen therapy, drug treatment and intravenous fluid infusion using life support in hazardous cases.

Coronavirus may demonstration of comparable proteins for virus reproduction in human immunodeficiency virus (HIV). Therefore, HIV protease inhibitors and nucleoside derivatives may be efficacious to treat COVID-19 like combination therapy of lopinavir. A minute ago, an Italian patient of COVID-19 is treated by making a combination of lopinavir (200 mg) and ritonavir (50 mg) twice a daytime, in Sawai Man Singh Hospital, Jaipur India. Equally well, the patient was also presented a combination of oseltamivir and chloroquine drug. The patient gets recovered and test was found negative for COVID-19. Some drugs are in clinical trial and outcomes are still expected. The best methodology to fight with viruses is vaccination. Consequently, scientists are trying to cultivate a vaccine for this virus and undoubtedly may be available later some time [7].

Remdesivir has effective in vitro activity against SARS-CoV-2, however, it is not US Food and Drug Administration permitted and presently is being tried out in continuing randomized trials. Corticosteroids are presently not recommended [8]. Existing clinical indication does not support to preventing angiotensin-converting enzyme inhibitors or angiotensin receptor blockers in patients with COVID-19. Some of the important class of drugs are listed below, which showing promising results as repurposed medicines in COVID-19 [9].

3.1. Antiviral Drugs

Drugs come under this category typically follow either of the next three mechanisms the ion channel blocking agent, virus-viral replication inhibition and serine protease inhibition. In market existing antiviral drugs typically target the four primary groups of viruses: herpes, hepatitis, human immunodeficiency virus and flu. Previous outbreak incidents of viral infections like SARS-CoV and MERS-CoV as well as haemorrhagic fever viruses like Ebola were manage with this category of drugs only [10, 11].

3.2. Antimalarial Drugs

It is comes under three groups grounded on their antifolate compound, mode of action aryl amino-alcohol compound and artemisinin. Maximum of these drugs are eradicated progressively from the body enduring for long periods of time after consumption. Disadvantage of this drugs are that antimalarial drug resistance cultivates for any drugs below this category [12, 13].

3.3. Anti-HIV Drugs

These drugs are categorised into diverse groups grounded on their targets retro-transcription, reverse transcription, viral-cell fusion, proteolytic processing, and combination of proviral DNA into the host genome and co-receptors interactions. Drugs comes under in these groups have been permitted by the Food and Drug Administration (FDA) and are nowadays publically used for the treatment of HIV.

3.4. Anti-Inflammatory Drugs

Enormous inflammatory response is detected in COVID- 19. Anti-inflammatory drugs, particularly JAK-STAT inhibitors are used in contradiction of rheumatoid arthritis, may be operational against raising levels of cytokines and valuable in preventing viral infection. Rendering to latest study, an inflammatory drug, baricitinib is when applied in combination by means of anti-viral drugs like Remidesivir, it increases the effectiveness of the drug to decrease viral infection [14, 15].

3.5. Monoclonal Antibodies

The virus is known to occur into the host cells by binding the S protein to ACE2 receptors. By emerging neutralizing antibodies in contradiction of the sense organs, there is a high probability for decreasing the harshness of the disease. Presently, only a few of drugs have been sanctioned for usage against SARS-CoV-2 [16].

3.6. Other Clinically Used Drugs

Even earlier the announcement of COVID-19 as a pandemic by WHO, there was an enormous lack of disease precise drugs. Due to promptly increasing virus, it is important to make available appropriate treatment for the affected patients. A list of possible drugs is providing in Table 1 and a few of the commonly used drugs are discussed below [17].

Table 1. Marketed allopathy drugs for the treatment of the COVID-19

Sr. No.	Drug Name	Disease Treated	References
1	Ritonavir + Lopinavir	MERS, SARS	[7]
2	Reverse Transcriptase inhibitor	SARS	[7]
3	Ribavirin	RSV pneumonia	[7, 25]
4	Alpha interferon	SARS and RSV	[7]
5	Cathespin L	SARS	[7]
6	Acyclovir	MERS, SARS and COVID-19	[7, 26]
7	Tocilizumab	COVID-19	[7]
8	Methylprednisolone	MERS, SARS	[7]
9	Thymosin alpha 1	MERS	[7]
10	Baloxavir marboxil	COVID-19	[7, 27]
11	Carfilzomib	COVID-19	[7]
12	Azvudine	COVID-19	[7]
13	Oseltamivir	COVID-19	[7]
14	Indinavir	COVID-19 and SARS	[1]
15	Saquinavir	SARS and Feline Coronavirus	[28]
16	Baricitinib	COVID-19	[29]
17	Ruxolitinib	COVID-19	[30]
18	ASC09	SARS and MERS ARDS	[31]

Table 1. (Continued)

Sr. No.	Drug Name	Disease Treated	References
19	Chloroquine	Coronavirus OC 43, SARS	[23, 32]
20	Alcohol inhalation therapy	COVID-19	[33]
21	Lopinavir	MERS and SARS, COVID-19	[34]
22	Darunavir	COVID-19	[35]
23	Favinavir	COVID-19	[36]
24	Remdesivir	MERS, SARS, COVID-19	[8]
25	Influenza drugs	MERS	[37]
26	Nitazoxanide	Influenza, MERS, and SARS	[38]
27	RNA dependent RNA Polymerase	Murine Coronavirus, SARS	[39]
28	Papain like protease	MERS and SARS	[40]
29	Umifenovir	Influenza, MERS and SARS	[35]
30	Fusion inhibitors i.e., Lamivudine adefovir dipivoxil etc.	SARS	[41]
31	Protease Inhibitors: saquinavir, ritonavir, indinavir, lopinavir etc	SARS	[42]
32	Nucleotide reverse transcriptase inhibitors: tenofovir disoproxil fumarate	SARS	[31]

3.6.1. Ribavirin

Ribavirin is one of the broad-spectrum drug whose therapeutic potential was revealed in 1972. This antiviral drug is used to treat hepatitis C. It is typically used with interferon α (IFN). This medicine is, approved by the USFDA, it plays for the active site of RdRp [18].

3.6.2. Sofosbuvir

This drug is also a FDA approved drug in contradiction of NS5B and target as a nucleotide polymerase inhibitor applied for the treatment of hepatitis C. It was applied in combination with interferon or RBV. This drug was earlier applied for the treatment of Zika virus [19].

3.6.3. Lopinavir/Ritonavir

Lopinavir/Ritonavir is a protease inhibitor, which objects the HIV virus. It was acknowledged by 1998 and approved by the USFDA by 2000. This drug blocks the formation of viral proteins by disturbing the proteolytic treating by mimicking its structure as a peptide cleaved by HIV protease. Ritonavir along with another flu drug, like oseltamivir was described to result in whole recovery after displaying signs of COVID-19 associated pneumonia [20].

3.6.4. Remidesivir (Anti-Viral Peptide)

This specific drug is an adenosine nucleotide analog, which was applied to treat in contradiction of SARS-CoV, MERS-CoV and Ebola [21]. It is a favourable and potential drug which roots premature cessation by entering the nascent viral RNA. Currently, it is undertaking clinical trials for Ebola treatment. Additional, recent study has showing that Remidesivir scored 0.77 μM at half maximal concentration beside COVID-19 and obstructed viral infection [22].

3.6.5. Chloroquine

This drug, comes under an anti-malarial drug, has exhibited potential in the treatment of avian influenza A. Chloroquine also has revealed potential to possess anti-viral and immune modulating properties. Chloroquine showed 1.13 μM at half maximal concentration in contradiction of SARS-CoV-2 and obstructed viral infection with increased in endosomal pH mandatory for viral fusion [23].

3.6.6. Favipiravir

It is a broad spectrum anti-viral drug which has got approval from Shenzan Health Commission for handling COVID–19 patients [24].

3.7. Other Ongoing Clinical Trials

Currently, there are numerous industries that have applied to clinical trials to repurpose of current drugs as well as to prepare vaccines and drugs to battle against the fast increasing COVID–19. In the situation of repurposing the available drugs, randomized controlled treatment (RCT) are being taken out by innumerable biotechnological enterprises as well as research institutes such as the National Institutes of Health (NIH), USA to recognize disease precise drugs. The use of repurposed medications relies on the supposition that the benefits (in vitro/clinical evidence) outweigh associated risks (adverse drug reactions). Overall, the rareness of evidence representing a clear advantage may not validate the risk of the repurposed drugs. This is of topmost distress in patients at high risk for toxicity and in this conditions were adverse measures may prevent entry into investigational trials [43, 44].

4. AYURVEDA

Indian traditional medical systems are well-thought-out as one of the ancient treatments in human history and it establishes a significant character in meeting worldwide health care essentials. Ancient Indian medical practices comprise Ayurveda, Unani, Siddha, Naturopathy, Homoeopathy and Yoga, which are productively used for treating numerous diseases. These patterns came into presence 5000 years before, and these systems have been observed and scripted in traditional literature. An ancient Indian medicine used minerals, plants and animal products for treating human illnesses. Traditional knowledge related to the plant roots and their applications are important to usage them precisely and for the proper circumstance. Around 25,000 plant centered preparations have been used in folk medications in, Indian medical history. A minute ago, the total total of Indian medicinal plants was measured to be around 3000, yet, traditional expert's usage nearby 8000 diverse species for their exercise. Traditional medicines are usually unnoticed in research and development of modern drugs, meanwhile their translational abilities are much underestimated. Even though these medicines are confusing, there are extensive contexts for their applications in non- Western medical technology [45]. A single plant may contain numerous phytochemical components that function alone or in combination with other constituents to produce the wanted pharmacological effect. Due to their applications in traditional medicine, numerous plant molecules have been studied and consequently moderated into drugs for several diseases. Searching for new compounds with antiviral activity has often been disappointing due to viral resistance laterally with viral latency and recurrent infection in immune compromised patients. Amongst antiviral therapeutic methods, the mainstream of them are non-specific for viruses, the progressions in increasing antiviral agents are the foremost focus in medical research. The antiviral properties of medicinal plants have established a fantastic role at various stages of viral development. Plant resulting pharmacological preparations marked a major influence for viral infections. Built on the availability of appropriate, effective and rapid bioassay systems, the antiviral compounds have been applied for prompt screening from plant extracts and fractions. In its home of synthetic antiviral drugs, medicinal plants bring basic raw materials for significant antiviral drugs. Synthetic drugs have been exchanged by medicinal plants, as life-saving drugs in numerous viral diseases. Unfortunately, the applications of these medicinal drugs have been handed down for generations by word of mouth and maximum of them have been missing over time, due to the absence of appropriate support. Investigation of these plants and medicinal herbs may help to endorse their applications in clinical settings to inhibit or treat different diseases. Later on many Indian medicinal herbs show antiviral, anti-inflammatory and antioxidant properties, it may be encouraging to consider them for the treatment of COVID-19. Some of them few significant medicinal plants are discussed infra.

Some investigations on coronavirus by means of medicinal plants are somewhat minimal in India, an investigation has shown anti-mouse coronaviral activity by the plants *Indigofera tinctoria (AO), Vitex trifolia, Abutilon indicum, Clerodendruminerme Gaertn, Leucas aspera, Cassia alata, Sphaeranthus indicus, Clitoriaternatea, Gymnema sylvestre, Pergulariadaemi and Evolvulus alsinoides* in Tamil Nadu. Amongst them Vitex trifolia and Sphaeranthus indicus have been set up to decrease inflammatory cytokines by means of the NF-kB pathway, a nerve tract that has been touched with the respiratory suffering in SARS-CoV. *Clitoris ternatea* has been recognised as a metalloproteinase inhibitor, ADAM17, a metalloproteinase that is involved in ACE destroying can be targeted applying this plant, as ACE-2 shredding has been associated with an augmented formation of viruses. The herbs Glycyrrhiza glabra and Allium sativum have been picked out to target the viral replication of SARS-CoV, rising as favourable candidates against SARS-CoV-2. *Clerodendrum inerme Gaertn,* another plant has been obtained to have the potential to deactivate the viral ribosome, this can be advance examined for its effectiveness as a drug targeting SARS-CoV-2 protein translation. Correspondingly, *Strobilanthes Cusia* blocked the viral RNA genome synthesis and encouraged pain like protease activity targeting the HCoV. In Asia, Himalayan forestry are plentifully flourishing with rich medicinal plant species and a study has recognized the presence of ethnomedicinal plants in contradiction of bronchitis. The invetigational screening of the antiviral herbs properties, in contrast to bronchitis, which exhibited that Hyoscyamus Niger, Justicia adhatoda and Verbascum thapsus decreased infections produced by flu viruses. The molecular mechanism by which these plants target an influenza virus can be deliberate to understand if they attack any molecules overlying between SARS-CoV-2 and the Influenza viruses. *Hyoscyamus Niger* was originated to be a bronchodilator and also had inhibitory effects on Ca2+ channel. This could be used to target the orf3a Ca2+channels that trigger numerous downstream pathways of viral infection. Maximum prominently, innumerable medicinal herbs have shown inhibitory properties contrary to ACE, and these comprise *Coriandrum sativum*, *Boerhaavia diffusa, Cynara scolymus, Coscinium fenestratum, Punicagranatum Cassia occidentalis* and *Embeliaribes*. Amongst them, Punicagranatum displayed a competitive style of action, although the sleep was non-specific inhibitors. These herbs required to be studied further to appear into their tangible effects on the entry of SARS-CoV-2 into the host cell. One of the most important species in the Acanthaceae family, *Andrographis paniculata* (kalmegh) existing in South Asia has a good treating ability of viral respiratory infections in Ayurvedic and other medicinal systems [46]. It was well-known that *Andrographis paniculata* suppressed improved NOD-like receptor protein 3 (NLRP3), caspase-1, and interleukin-1β molecules which are expansively take part in the pathogenesis of SARS-COV and likely SARS-CoV-2 as well. *Salacia oblonga* another herb from Tamil Nadu has also showed suppressive properties on angiotensin II, AT1 signal, which was associated to lung damage. Numerous herbs have also showing inhibitory response towards HIV proteases, these herbs can be auspicious drugs for COVID-19. They comprise, *Acacia nilotica, Eugenia jambolana, Euphorbia granulate*. Some herbs like *Ocimum sanctum, Ocimumkilim and scharicum, Solanum nigrum, Vitex negundo[47]* have been well known to target the reverse transcriptase action of HIV and can be investigated for activity in contradiction of SARS-CoV-2 as well. More, *Sambucus ebulus* has been recognised to inhibit the activity of enclosed viruses and can also be applied to target this virus. These medicinal herbs can be applied to ameliorate the symptoms of COVID-19 [48]. Although numerous medicinal herbs have been recognised, a lot of investigation has to be carried out for the development of drug precise to SARS-CoV-2. Consequently, it is significant to discover the result of these recommended traditional medicines on SARS-CoV-2 [49, 50].

5. Unani Medicines

Unani method of medicinal treatment also the based on the plant and associated stuffs. The various portions of the numerous herbs are well known for a long time for their anti-viral properties. The utmost significant herbs are Glycyrrhiza glabra, Allium cepa, Allium sativum, Ocimum sanctum, Ocimum tenuiflorum, Piper nigrum, Cinnamomum verum, Daucus Mauritius, Curcuma longa, etc. An aqueous infusion of these herbaceous plants along with lemon juice or honey was found to be operative for the flu and common cold virus contaminations.s contaminations. The utmost significant herbs are Glycyrrhiza glabra, Allium cepa, Allium sativum, Ocimum sanctum, Ocimum tenuiflorum, Piper nigrum, Cinnamomum verum, Daucus Mauritius, Curcuma longa, etc. An aqueous infusion of these herbaceous plants along with lemon juice or honey was found to be operative for the flu and common cold virus contaminations. The root of Licorice (Glycyrrhiza glabra) is easily known to possess a good antiviral activity. This plant is observed in Asia and Europe and documented as a weed. Fiore et al. (2008) carried out an *in vitro* investigation of *Glycyrrhiza glabra* plant and stated that this plant displayed antiviral properties of different viruses comprising SARS associated coronavirus, HIV-1, and respiratory syncytial virus [51]. A review of the antiviral activity of *Glycyrrhiza glabra*. They are reported this plant active in contradiction of SARS, HIV, varicella zoster, hepatitis A, B, C, cytomegalo virus herpes simplex type-1. One more review was on the antiviral properties of the Glycyrrhiza glabra plant. Authors designated the properties of this plant contrary to various viruses like H1N1, H5N1, Influenza A virus (IAV), Hepatitis C virus, Rotavirus, HIV and SARS-associated coronavirus. Similarly, one reported a follow-up of the antiviral and antimicrobial properties of Glycyrrhiza glabra. Authors reported the existence of more than 300 flavonoids and 20 triterpenoids in this herb [52]. Authors also concise the active constituents and the greatest possible mechanisms of these above may be applicable to control COVID-19. This, January 29, 2020, the Government of India allotted an advisory constructed on Indian traditional medicine practices Ayurveda, Homeopathy and Unani, New Delhi. It comprises the methods of preventive management and designated a list of few Unani medicaments [53, 54].

6. Homeopathy

With regards homeopathy, arsenic at very small concentration is measured helpful for numerous diseases comprising viral infections. A moment ago, Directorate of AYUSH, New Delhi, India distributed an order dater on January 30, 2020, to take prophylactic medicine to evade coronavirus infection. The directorate recommended taking 4 pills of Arsenic Album-30 medicine per day in empty stomach for 3 days [55]. Arsenic Album-30 is extremely diluted arsenic trioxide and applicable as homeopathic prophylaxis. It is important to note here that there is no clinical confirmation for Arsenic Album-30 medicament as an operative medicine. Afterward that, a criticism for homeopathy came into being and it was known as pseudoscience [56]. An article is available in Taiwan Medical News on February, 2020 (https://www.thailandmedical.news/news/india-slammedfor-proposing-usage-of-homeopathy-to-prevent-coronavirus) and some people complained homeopathy to manage COVID-19 infection. The individuals who criticized most are Dr. David Robert Grimes and Dr. Edzard Ernst (Irish science write and an emeritus professor, University of Exeter, UK and a critic of homeopathy). Though, Dr. Mitchell Fleisher (vice president, American Institute of Homeopathy) recommended to transport away a relative clinical study on the acute coronavirus infection by giving to homeopathic medications to the patents and the experimental group, and allopathic medicines to another group, for 250 patients in each group. It was highly criticized it as completely unethical and as per to him, Homeopathy has no judicious mechanism of activity. Additionally, he added that it is unreliable to suggest a trial for a thoughtful pandemic [57]. They also let out that numerous investigations on homeopathy have designated that it does not operate. Also, the news director of Thailand Medical News Jakkapong Watcharachaijunta complained the use of homeopathic medicine in regulating COVID-19. At this conclusion, it is really significant to declaring the work of Dr. Robert T. Mathie (2013) whose research work designated that Arsenic album medicine as an operative to decrease fever, runny nose, headache, sore throat in the patients with swine influenza symptoms. Moreover, it experienced that some homeopathic medicines are operative to treat a diversity of diseases [57].

7. Other Immune System Boosters

It is witnessed that primary deaths were in older people, perhaps since of the poor immunity, which nurtures faster progress of COVID-19. Consequently, it is important to increase our immune system. It is significant to recommend that people should use some supplements to improve their immune systems [58]. Fit people should take sufficiently of citrus fruits having numerous vitamins. Some dry fruits (almonds, walnuts, and dates) are also valuable to increase the immune system. Nonetheless, elder people and the patients may take vitamins and zinc supplements with the discussion of medical practitioners. The significant vitamins are A, C, D and E. It is also worthwhile to take zinc and iodine intakes. It is also wise not to smoke and avoid any stress and do appropriate and regular workouts [59, 60].

Conclusion

Nevertheless, prevention and management are the best options till for the COVID-19. Different combination of drugs may be the best choice to treat the patients, on the basis of the patient's circumstances and symptoms. Though, Ayurveda and Unani therapy may be measured along with allopathic treatment. Perchance, the number of COVID-19 cases may lose weight in the coming time and the pace of virus spread may be depressed. It was realized that this disease is spread amongst those who are not considering it badly. So, above discussed different therapies will plays an important character to control the pandemic till the specific and effective medication and vaccine will not hear. Besides, there is an urgent necessity to identify novel therapies by using this type of different medical schemes. It is also really important to develop our young genesis of science and technology to fight in contradiction of any such tragedy in the hereafter; if any.

Acknowledgments

Authors are thankful to the Divine Collage of Pharmacy, Satana for providing facilities and the encouragement to write this chapter.

CONFLICT OF INTEREST

The authors declare that no conflict of interest.

REFERENCES

[1] Dong, L., S. Hu, and J. Gao, Discovering drugs to treat coronavirus disease 2019 (COVID-19). *Drug discoveries & therapeutics,* 2020. 14(1): p. 58-60.

[2] Singhal, T., A review of coronavirus disease-2019 (COVID-19). *The Indian Journal of Pediatrics,* 2020: p. 1-6.

[3] Cascella, M., et al., *Features, evaluation and treatment coronavirus (COVID-19),* in Statpearls [internet]. 2020, StatPearls Publishing.

[4] Zumla, A., et al., Reducing mortality from 2019-nCoV: host-directed therapies should be an option. *The Lancet,* 2020. 395(10224): p. e35-e36.

[5] Jin, Y.-H., et al., A rapid advice guideline for the diagnosis and treatment of 2019 novel coronavirus (2019-nCoV) infected pneumonia (standard version). *Military Medical Research,* 2020. 7(1): p. 4.

[6] Organization, W. H., *Coronavirus disease 2019 (COVID-19): situation report*, 73. 2020.

[7] Ali, I. and O. M. Alharbi, COVID-19: Disease, management, treatment, and social impact. *Science of the Total Environment,* 2020: p. 138861.

[8] Wang, Y., et al., Remdesivir in adults with severe COVID-19: a randomised, double-blind, placebo-controlled, multicentre trial. *The Lancet,* 2020.

[9] Al-Tawfiq, J. A., A. H. Al-Homoud, and Z. A. Memish, Remdesivir as a possible therapeutic option for the COVID-19. *Travel medicine and infectious disease,* 2020.

[10] Mitjà, O. and B. Clotet, Use of antiviral drugs to reduce COVID-19 transmission. *The Lancet Global Health,* 2020. 8(5): p. e639-e640.

[11] Gautret, P., et al., Hydroxychloroquine and azithromycin as a treatment of COVID-19: results of an open-label non-randomized clinical trial. *International journal of antimicrobial agents,* 2020: p. 105949.

[12] Jaffe, S., Regulators split on antimalarials for COVID-19. *The Lancet,* 2020. 395(10231): p. 1179.

[13] Touret, F. and X. de Lamballerie, of chloroquine and COVID-19. *Antiviral research,* 2020: p. 104762.

[14] Zhang, W., et al., The use of anti-inflammatory drugs in the treatment of people with severe coronavirus disease 2019 (COVID-19): The experience of clinical immunologists from China. *Clinical Immunology,* 2020: p. 108393.

[15] Cao, X., COVID-19: immunopathology and its implications for therapy. *Nature reviews immunology,* 2020. 20(5): p. 269-270.

[16] Shanmugaraj, B., et al., Perspectives on monoclonal antibody therapy as potential therapeutic intervention for Coronavirus disease-19 (COVID-19). *Asian Pac J Allergy Immunol,* 2020. 38(1): p. 10-18.

[17] Smith, T. and T. Prosser, COVID-19 Drug Therapy–Potential Options, in Clinical Drug Information, Clinical Solutions, Elsevier. Retrieved on Mar 16, 2020. 2020.

[18] Khalili, J. S., et al., Novel coronavirus treatment with ribavirin: Groundwork for an evaluation concerning COVID-19. *Journal of medical virology,* 2020.

[19] Elfiky, A. A., Ribavirin, Remdesivir, Sofosbuvir, Galidesivir, and Tenofovir against SARS-CoV-2 RNA dependent RNA polymerase (RdRp): A molecular docking study. *Life sciences,* 2020: p. 117592.

[20] Lim, J., et al., Case of the index patient who caused tertiary transmission of COVID-19 infection in Korea: the application of lopinavir/ritonavir for the treatment of COVID-19 infected pneumonia monitored by quantitative RT-PCR. *Journal of Korean medical science,* 2020. 35(6).

[21] Grein, J., et al., Compassionate use of remdesivir for patients with severe Covid-19. *New England Journal of Medicine,* 2020.

[22] Beigel, J. H., et al., Remdesivir for the treatment of Covid-19—preliminary report. *New England Journal of Medicine,* 2020.

[23] Colson, P., et al., Chloroquine and hydroxychloroquine as available weapons to fight COVID-19. *Int J Antimicrob Agents,* 2020. 105932(10.1016).

[24] Du, Y. X. and X. P. Chen, Favipiravir: pharmacokinetics and concerns about clinical trials for 2019-nCoV infection. *Clinical Pharmacology & Therapeutics,* 2020.

[25] Hung, I. F. N., et al., Triple combination of interferon beta-1b, lopinavir–ritonavir, and ribavirin in the treatment of patients admitted to hospital with COVID-19: an open-label, randomised, phase 2 trial. *The Lancet,* 2020. 395(10238): p. 1695-1704.

[26] Scavone, C., et al., Current pharmacological treatments for COVID-19: what's next? *British Journal of Pharmacology,* 2020.

[27] Lou, Y., L. Liu, and Y. Qiu, Clinical Outcomes and Plasma Concentrations of Baloxavir Marboxil and Favipiravir in COVID-19 Patients: an Exploratory Randomized, Controlled Trial. *medRxiv,* 2020.

[28] Pant, S., et al., Peptide-like and small-molecule inhibitors against Covid-19. *Journal of Biomolecular Structure and Dynamics,* 2020(just-accepted): p. 1-15.

[29] Favalli, E. G., et al., Baricitinib for COVID-19: a suitable treatment? *The Lancet Infectious Diseases,* 2020.

[30] Blanco-Melo, D., et al., Imbalanced host response to SARS-CoV-2 drives development of COVID-19. Cell, 2020.

[31] Zhai, P., et al., The epidemiology, diagnosis and treatment of COVID-19. *International journal of antimicrobial agents,* 2020: p. 105955.

[32] Cortegiani, A., et al., A systematic review on the efficacy and safety of chloroquine for the treatment of COVID-19. *Journal of critical care,* 2020.

[33] Cao, Y., Suggestion Using Alcohol Vaporization or Nebulization Inhalation Therapy for Pneumonitis Caused by Coronavirus. Available at SSRN 3545744, 2020.

[34] Yao, T. T., et al., A systematic review of lopinavir therapy for SARS coronavirus and MERS coronavirus—A possible reference for coronavirus disease-19 treatment option. *Journal of medical virology,* 2020. 92(6): p. 556-563.

[35] Costanzo, M., M. A. R. De Giglio, and G. N. Roviello, SARS-CoV-2: recent reports on antiviral therapies based on lopinavir/ritonavir, darunavir/umifenovir, hydroxychloroquine, remdesivir, favipiravir and other drugs for the treatment of the new coronavirus. *Current medicinal chemistry,* 2020.

[36] Abdul Kadhim, A., N. Hadi, and M. Abdulhussein, Preprocessing of the Candidate Antiviral Drugs against COVID-19 in Models of SARS cov2 Targets. *Prensa Med Argent,* 2020. 106: p. 2.

[37] Chen, J., et al., Clinical study of mesenchymal stem cell treating acute respiratory distress syndrome induced by epidemic Influenza A (H7N9) infection, a hint for COVID-19 treatment. *Engineering,* 2020.

[38] Srivatsan Padmanabhan, M., *Potential dual therapeutic approach against SARS-CoV-2/COVID-19 with Nitazoxanide and Hydroxychloroquine.*

[39] Gao, Y., et al., Structure of the RNA-dependent RNA polymerase from COVID-19 virus. *Science,* 2020. 368(6492): p. 779-782.

[40] Arya, R., et al., *Potential inhibitors against papain-like protease of novel coronavirus (SARS-CoV-2) from FDA approved drugs*. 2020.

[41] Iyer, M., et al., COVID-19: an update on diagnostic and therapeutic approaches. *BMB reports,* 2020. 53(4): p. 191.

[42] Boopathi, S., A.B. Poma, and P. Kolandaivel, Novel 2019 coronavirus structure, mechanism of action, antiviral drug promises and rule out against its treatment. *Journal of Biomolecular Structure and Dynamics,* 2020(just-accepted): p. 1-14.

[43] Lythgoe, M. P. and P. Middleton, Ongoing clinical trials for the management of the COVID-19 pandemic. *Trends in Pharmacological Sciences,* 2020.

[44] Kalil, A. C., Treating COVID-19—off-label drug use, compassionate use, and randomized clinical trials during pandemics. *Jama,* 2020. 323(19): p. 1897-1898.

[45] Golechha, M., Time to realise the true potential of Ayurveda against COVID-19. *Brain, Behavior, and Immunity,* 2020.

[46] Patwardhan, B., et al., Ayurveda rasayana in prophylaxis of covid-19. *Curr Sci,* 2020. 118: p. 1158-1160.

[47] Goothy, S. S. K., et al., Ayurveda's Holistic Lifestyle Approach for the Management of Coronavirus disease (COVID-19): Possible Role of Tulsi. *International Journal of Research in Pharmaceutical Sciences,* 2020. 11(SPL1): p. 16-18.

[48] Balkrishna, A., *Indian Traditional Ayurvedic Treatment Regime For Novel Coronavirus, COVID-19.*

[49] Rajkumar, R. P., Ayurveda and COVID-19: where psycho-neuroimmunology and the meaning response meet. *Brain, Behavior, and Immunity,* 2020.

[50] Prarthana, H., S. S. Kokatnur, and S. Desai, Understanding of Covid-19 disease through Ayurveda. *Journal of Ayurveda and Integrated Medical Sciences* (ISSN 2456-3110), 2020. 5(2): p. 169-174.

[51] Nikhat, S. and M. Fazil, Overview of Covid-19; its prevention and management in the light of Unani medicine. *Science of The Total Environment,* 2020: p. 138859.

[52] Hashmi, D. and S. Mujtabaali, Broad Spectrum Antiviral Prophylactic Medicine (Unani) to Induce Immunity and Heard Immunity to Prevent the Spread of Novel Corona Virus. *Broad Spectrum Antiviral Prophylactic Medicine (Unani) to Induce Immunity and Heard Immunity to Prevent the Spread of Novel Corona Virus* (May 5, 2020), 2020.

[53] Chaturvedi, S., et al., Ayush, modern medicine and the Covid-19 pandemic. *Indian Jour Med Ethics*, 2020.

[54] Priya, R. and V. Sujatha, AYUSH for COVID-19: Science or Superstition? *Indian Journal of Public Health,* 2020. 64(6): p. 105.

[55] Chaudhary, A. and A. Khurana, A review on the role of Homoeopathy in epidemics with some reflections on COVID-19 (SARS-CoV-2). *Indian Journal of Research in Homoeopathy,* 2020. 14(2): p. 100.

[56] Azis, S. P. and H. Kaur, Enabling use of Homoeopathy in India's preparedness for pandemic/epidemic situation like COVID-19. *Indian Journal of Research in Homoeopathy,* 2020. 14(2): p. 143.

[57] Parikh, N. and D. Parikh, Role of homoeopathy in COVID-19 Management-A clinical experience. *World J. Pharm. Res,* 2020. 9(5): p. 2459.

[58] Jawhara, S., Could Intravenous immunoglobulin collected from recovered coronavirus patients protect against COVID-19 and strengthen the immune system of new patients? *International journal of molecular sciences,* 2020. 21(7): p. 2272.

[59] Doss, M., *Treatment of COVID-19 with Individualized Immune Boosting Interventions*. 2020.

[60] Shi, Y., et al., *COVID-19 infection: the perspectives on immune responses.* 2020, Nature Publishing Group.

In: COVID-19 Pandemic
Editor: A. K. Haghi
ISBN: 978-1-53618-565-2

Chapter 3

FLU, SYPHILIS, HIV, HEPATITIS, VIRUS EVOLUTION, CORONAVIRUS AND DENGUE

***Francisco Torrens*[1,*] *and Gloria Castellano*[2]**
[1]Institut Universitari de Ciència Molecular, Universitat de València, Edifici d'Instituts de Paterna, València, Spain
[2]Departamento de Ciencias Experimentales y Matemáticas, Facultad de Veterinaria y Ciencias Experimentales, Universidad Católica de Valencia San Vicente Mártir, Guillem de Castro-94, València, Spain

ABSTRACT

This review concerns to the *filling* of peeps concerning a topic. The thoughts *result previously mingling*, and the job is to allow contact. One does not discontinue meeting his long-established doubts once reasoning about the condition, *via* the optics of the *condition of exclusion* and an administration that controls liberties in the name of safety. One more proposes that the disaster will compel persons to reason in a different society, outside the country condition, and they should *recreate collectivism founded on faith in persons and in knowledge*; i.e., every

* Corresponding Author's E-mail: torrens@uv.es.

specialist carries water to his own mill, and *utilizes* the present disaster to settle the tragedies that his philosophies previously forecasted or endorse the kind of administration he wishes. A tad in the design of a *novel stage* self-support monograph, this revision pursues to twist to the specialists, as if they resulted a mystical teacher able to light the trail that aids persons outdoors the dim cave, in which they abruptly understood they resulted continuously isolated. Specialists result admonished for appearing to hypothesise beforehand on a disaster that persons are not able up till now to understand, owing to the excellent character of the condition.

Keywords: RNA virus, viroid, RNA secondary structure, phylogenetics, flu-transmission multi-scale modelling; Intervention evaluation, genetic study

1. Introduction

Setting the scene: multi-scale modelling for the transmission of influenza, the evaluation of interventions towards it, the origin of modern syphilis, the emergence of a pandemic *Treponema pallidum* cluster, the molecular epidemiology of human immunodeficiency virus (HIV) type 1 (-1) in the Valencian Community (VC, Spain), the analysis of transmission clusters, the effect of ribonucleic acid (RNA) substitution models on viroid, RNA virus phylogenies, host factors in coronavirus (CoV) replication, using paired serology and surveillance data to quantify dengue transmission and control during a large outbreak in Fiji, and complexities of epidemics.

Severe acute respiratory syndrome (SARS)-CoV is an agent of emerging and reemerging infection [1]. Global shifts in mammalian population trends revealed key predictors of virus spillover risk [2]. The proximal origin of SARS-CoV clade 2 (SARS-CoV-2) was proposed [3]. An interactive web-based dashboard to track CoV disease 2019 (COVID-19) in real time (RT) was designed [4]. Mas-Coma group informed COVID-19 and globalization [5]. They reported coalition as advocacy for prospective clinical trials (CTs) to test the post-exposure potential of hydroxychloroquine against COVID-19 [6]. Galvez group reported drugs repurposing for CoV treatment as a computational study based on molecular topology [7]. Can a virus undermine human rights [8]? People must answer the right questions for policymakers on COVID-19 [9]. Trust must be built while influencing online COVID-19 content in the social media world [10]. Ethnicity in COVID-19 must be an urgent public health (PH) research priority [11]. A modelling study nowcasted and forecasted the potential domestic and international spread of the SARS-CoV-2 outbreak originating in Wuhan, China [12]. Offline, COVID-19 and the NHS were proposed as *a national scandal* [13]. In the novel CoV outbreak, what people know and what they do not were presented [14]. The COVID-19 as navigating uncertainties together was discussed [15]. The COVID-19 is a data science issue [16]. Countries must differentiate COVID-19 response strategies [17]. Viral entry of SARS-CoV-2 is mediated *via* viral spike protein and host ACE2 enzyme interaction. [18]. Imbalanced host response to SARS-CoV-2 drives development of COVID-19 [19]. A multibasic cleavage site in the spike protein of SARS-CoV-2 is essential for infection of human lung cells [20]. Receptor ACE2 of SARS-CoV-2 is an interferon-stimulated gene in human airway epithelial cells and is detected in specific cell subsets across tissues [21]. Full-genome evolutionary analysis of SARS-CoV-2 rejects the hypothesis of emergence as a result of a recent recombination event [22]. Pathogenicity and transmissibility of SARS-CoV-2 were studied *via* a quick overview and comparison with other emerging viruses [23]. The SARS-CoV-2, COVID-19, the epidemic and the challenges were informed [24]. Insights into the recent novel SARS-CoV-2 in light of past human CoV outbreaks were reviewed [25]. Insight into 2019 novel CoV was revised with an updated interim review with lessons from SARS-CoV and Middle East respiratory syndrome (MERS)-CoV [26]. Sex-bias in COVID-19 was meta-analysed and reviewed based on sex differences in disease and immunity [27]. The COVID-19 evolves in human hosts [28]. The COVID-19 is a lesson in humility, and an opportunity for sagacity and hope [29]. COVID-19: The isolation that has brought us together [30]. An RT dashboard of CTs for

COVID-19 was informed [31]. COVID-19 is a new virus, but a familiar receptor and cytokine release syndrome [32].

In the present report, it was reviewed multi-scale modelling for the transmission of influenza, the evaluation of interventions towards it, the origin of modern syphilis, the emergence of a pandemic *Treponema pallidum* cluster, the molecular epidemiology of HIV-1 in the VC (Spain), the analysis of transmission clusters, the effect of RNA substitution models on viroid, RNA virus phylogenies, host factors in CoV replication, using paired serology and surveillance data to quantify dengue transmission and control during a large outbreak in Fiji, and complexities of epidemics.

2. Flu-Transmission Multi-Scale Modelling: Evaluation of Interventions

Mathematical modelling of influenza epidemic is important for analyzing the main cause of the epidemic and finding effective interventions to it. The epidemic is a dynamic process, in which daily infections are caused by people's contacts, and the frequency of contacts can be mainly influenced by their cognition to the disease. The cognition is in turn influenced by daily illness attack rate, climate, and other environment factors. Few existing methods considered the dynamic process in their models. Their prediction results can hardly be explained by the mechanisms of epidemic spreading. A heterogeneous graph modelling (HGM) was developed to describe the dynamic process of influenza virus transmission, taking advantage of unique clinical data [33]. Social net of studied region was built, and an agent-based model was embedded in HGM to describe the dynamic change of an epidemic. The simulations present a good agreement with clinical data. Parameter sensitivity analysis showed that temperature influences the dynamic of epidemic significantly and system behaviour analysis showed social net degree is a critical factor determining the size of an epidemic. Multiple scenarios for vaccination and school closure strategies were simulated, and their performance was analyzed.

3. A Genetic Study that Fixes the Origin of the Syphilis Bacterium

The abrupt onslaught of the syphilis pandemic that started in the late 15th century established the devastating infectious disease as one of the most feared in human history. Surprisingly, despite the availability of effective antibiotic treatment since the mid-20th century, the bacterial infection, which is caused by *Treponema pallidum* subsp. *pallidum* (TPA), was re-emerging globally in the last few decades with 10 600 000 cases in 2008. Although resistance to penicillin is not identified, an increasing number of strains fail to respond to the second-line antibiotic azithromycin. Little is known about the genetic patterns in current infections or the evolutionary origins of the disease because of the low quantities of treponemal deoxyribonucleic acid (DNA) in clinical samples and difficulties in cultivating the pathogen. Capture of DNA and whole-genome sequencing were used to interrogate successfully genome-wide variation from syphilis patient specimens, combined with TPA laboratory samples and two other subspecies [34]. Phylogenetic comparisons based on the sequenced genomes indicate that the examined TPA strains share a common ancestor after the 15th century, in the early modern era. Most contemporary strains are azithromycin-resistant and members of a globally dominant cluster (SS14-Ω). The cluster diversified from a common ancestor in the mid-20th century subsequent to the discovery of antibiotics. Its recent phylogenetic divergence and global presence point to the emergence of a pandemic strain cluster.

4. Characterizing Dynamics of HIV Transmission in Valencian Community

Infections of HIV are a serious concern for PH worldwide. Molecular evolution was applied to study HIV-1 epidemics in VC (Spain) from a PH surveillance perspective [35]. For this, 1 804 HIV-1 sequences comprising protease and reverse transcriptase (PR/RT) coding regions were analysed, sampled in 2004-2014, which sequences were subtyped and subjected to phylogenetic analyses in order to detect transmission clusters. Univariate and multinomial comparisons were performed to detect epidemiological differences between HIV-1 subtypes, and risk groups. The HIV epidemic in VC is dominated by subtype-B infections among local men who have sex with men (MSM). A total of 270 transmission clusters were identified (> 57% of the dataset), 12 of which included ≥10 patients; 11 of subtype B (9 affecting MSMs) and one (n = 21) of CRF14, affecting predominately intravenous drug users (IDUs). Dated phylogenies revealed the large clusters to have originated from the mid-1980s to the early 2000s. Subtype B is more likely to form transmission clusters than non-B variants, and MSMs, to cluster than other risk groups. Multinomial analyses revealed an association between non-B variants, which are not established in the local population, and different foreign groups.

5. Reconstructing Evolution of Aids, Hepatitis and Influenza Viruses

Many viroids and RNA viruses present genomes that exhibit secondary structure, with paired nucleotides forming stems and loops. Such structures violate a key assumption of most methods of phylogenetic reconstruction: that sequence change is independent among sites. However, phylogenetic analyses of the transmissible agents rarely use evolutionary models that account for RNA secondary structure. The effect of using RNA-specific nucleotide substitution models on the phylogenetic inference of viroids and RNA viruses was assessed [36]. Datasets comprising full-genome nucleotide sequences from six viroid and 10 single-stranded RNA virus species were obtained. For each alignment, consensus RNA secondary structures were inferred, then different DNA and RNA substitution models were evaluated. Model selection was used to choose the best-fitting model and evaluate estimated Bayesian phylogenies. For each dataset, Robinson–

Foulds (RF) statistics were generated and compared, in order to test whether the distributions of trees generated under alternative models are notably different to each other. In all alignments, the best-fitting model was one that considers RNA secondary structure: RNA models that allow a nonzero rate of double substitution (RNA16A, RNA16C) fitted the best for viral and viroid datasets. In 14 of 16 datasets, the use of an RNA-specific model led to significantly longer tree lengths, but only in three cases it presented a significant effect on RFs. In conclusion, *via* RNA model when undertaking phylogenetic inference of viroids and RNA viruses could provide a better model fit than standard approaches, and model choice could significantly affect branch length estimates.

6. Host Factors in Coronavirus Replication

The CoVs are pathogens with a serious impact on human and animal health. They mostly cause enteric or respiratory disease, which can be severe and life threatening, e.g., in the case of the zoonotic CoVs causing SARS and MERS in humans. In spite of the economic and societal impact of such CoV infections, and the likelihood of future outbreaks of additional pathogenic CoVs, people's options to prevent or treat CoV infections remain limited, which highlights the importance of advancing their knowledge on the replication of the viruses and their interactions with the host. Compared to other positive stranded (+)RNA viruses, CoVs present an exceptionally large genome and employ a complex genome expression strategy. Next to a role in basic virus replication or virus assembly, many CoV proteins expressed in the infected cell contribute to CoV-host interplay; e.g., interacting with the host cell to create an optimal environment for CoV replication, altering host gene expression or counteracting the host's antiviral defenses. The CoV–host interactions are key to viral pathogenesis and will determine the outcome of infection. Because of the complexity of the CoV proteome and replication cycle, people's knowledge of host factors involved in CoV replication is still in an early stage compared to what is known for other +RNA viruses. Current understanding of CoV–host interactions at the level of the infected cell was reviewed, with special attention for the assembly and function of the viral RNA-synthesising machinery and the evasion of cellular innate immune responses [37]. The surface spike (S) glycoprotein is critical for binding of host cell receptors and is believed to represent a key determinant of host range restriction [38].

7. Serology/Surveillance to Quantify Dengue Transmission and Control

Dengue is a major health burden, but it can be challenging to examine transmission and evaluate control measures because outbreaks depend on multiple factors (e.g., human population structure, prior immunity, climate). Population-representative paired sera collected before and after 2013/14 dengue-3 outbreak in Fiji were combined with surveillance data, in order to determine how such factors influence transmission and control in island settings [39]. The results showed the 10–19 year-old age group had the highest risk of infection, but strong evidence was not find that other demographic or environmental risk factors were linked to seroconversion. A mathematical model jointly fitted to surveillance and serological data showed that herd immunity and seasonally varying transmission could not explain observed dynamics. However, the model showed evidence of an additional reduction in transmission coinciding with a vector clean-up campaign, which may have contributed to the decline in cases in the later stages of the outbreak. Exasperated many people are by governments' response to COVID-19, such decisions are ultimately political. People must hold politicians to account for PH shortcomings, and recognise and value the complex specialist work that disease modellers undertake. *The Rules of Contagion* is a timely reminder of the importance of disease modelling [40]. Without such models, people would be in far greater trouble battling COVID-19 [41].

8. Complexities of Epidemics

As epidemics evolve, all factors are interacting, and the entire web of humanity and human organizations are individually and collectively reacting to the situation around them [42]. In the case of Ebola, a single case that occurred in a Texas Hospital lead to people avoiding going to that hospital for any reason, even if no direct risk existed to them, and turning the hospital into a virtual ghost town. In the midst of epidemics, people and organizations are taking cues from each other and taking cues from the data as they become available. The complexities of the multiple factors at play in rapidly moving large scale events make a honed and practiced general preparedness process essential. The underlying preparedness framework is what allows solutions and consensus emerge. However, when so many factors are moving at such a rapid pace, the *perfect response* seems elusive (in part because the definition of success would be to have never suffering or mortality from an epidemic to begin with). The potential number of failure points result numerous, and success can usually be assessed in only retrospect.

9. Discussion

The epidemic presents many variables [43]. However, four letters are key (DOTS):

D, duration;
O, opportunity:
T, transmissibility;
S, susceptibility.

By lowering the opportunity, people will be able to stop the curve of the epidemic.

CONCLUSION

From the present results and discussion, the following final remarks can be drawn:

1. Finding the best way to prevent an epidemic is a challenging task because interactions between individuals are highly connected and complicated in today's world. Net modeling results a flexible tool to build a plausible world, to re-enact past epidemics and simulate future outbreaks, and to analyze the major causes leading to spread of the disease.
2. Genomic diversity of *T. pallidum* subsp. *pallidum* was examined from syphilis samples isolated during 20/21st centuries. The first reported whole genome sequences successfully obtained directly from syphilis patients were reported. The analyses indicate that all *T. p. pallidum* samples share a common ancestor that was infecting populations in the early centuries of the modern era.
3. Human immunodeficiency virus type-1 epidemic in Comunitat Valenciana is dominated by subtype B, especially among local men who have sex with men. Although an important number of non-B cases existed, they occurred mostly among immigrants, which shows that non-B infections are not well established in the local population. However, the detection of transmission clusters of non-B variants urges to increase efforts on human immunodeficiency virus testing.
4. Previous phylogenetic analyses of viral and viroid genomes were undertaken *via* deoxyribonucleic-acid substitution models. However, in the light of the results, such analyses should consider the inclusion of ribonucleic-acid models, as they may better describe the evolution of paired sites.
5. Despite the caveats, the results show that transmission dynamic models developed *via* a combination of serological surveys and surveillance data are a valuable tool for examining dengue fever outbreaks. As well as providing insights into the transmission and

control of dengue, the analysis presents implications for forecasting of future epidemics.

6. By lowering the opportunity, people will be able to stop the curve of the epidemic. Learning from history is essential even though they cannot prevent pathogens' natural evolution.

ACKNOWLEDGMENTS

The authors acknowledge Dr. Vicente Simón by the online courses *Mindfulness in Times of Crisis* and financial support from Fundación Universidad Católica de Valencia *San Vicente Mártir* (Project No. 2019-217-001UCV).

REFERENCES

[1] Cheng, VCC; Lau, SKP; Woo, PCY; Yuen, KY. Severe acute respiratory syndrome coronavirus as an agent of emerging and reemerging infection. *Clin. Microbiol. Rev.*, 2007, 20, 660-694.

[2] Johnson, CK; Hitchens, PL; Pandit, PS; Rushmore, J; Evans, TS; Young, CCW; Doyle, MM. Global shifts in mammalian population trends reveal key predictors of virus spillover risk. *Proc. R. Soc. B*, 2020, 287, 2736–1-10.

[3] Andersen, KG; Rambaut, A; Lipkin, WI; Holmes, EC; Garry, RF. The proximal origin of SARS-CoV-2. *Nat. Med.*, 2020, 26, 450-452.

[4] Dong, E; Du, H; Gardner, L. An interactive web-based dashboard to track COVID-19 in real time. *Lancet Infect. Dis.*, 2020, 30120-1, 1-2.

[5] Mas-Coma, S; Jones, MK; Marty, AM. COVID-19 and globalization. *One Health* 2020, 9, 100132–1-4.

[6] Picot, S; Marty, A; Bienvenu, AL; Blumberg, LH; Dupouy-Camet, J; Carnevale, P; Kano, S; Jones, MK; Daniel-Ribeiro, CT; Mas-Coma, S. Coalition: Advocacy for prospective clinical trials to test the post-

exposure potential of hydroxychloroquine against COVID-19. *One Health*, 2020, 9, 100131–1-5.

[7] Galvez, J; Zanni, R; Galvez-Llompart, M. Drugs repurposing for coronavirus treatment: Computational study based on molecular topology. *Nereis*, 2020, 2020(12), 15-18.

[8] *Nay, O.* Can a virus undermine human rights? *Lancet Public Health*, 2020, 30092-X, 1-2.

[9] Graeden, E; Carlson, C; Katz, *R.* Answering the right questions for policymakers on COVID-19. *Lancet Glob. Health*, 2020, 30191-1, 1-2.

[10] Limaye, RJ; Sauer, M; Ali, J; Bernstein, J; Wahl, B; Barnhill, A; Labrique, A. Building trust while influencing online COVID-19 content in the social media world. *Lancet Dig. Health*, 2020, 30084–4, 1-2.

[11] Pareek, M; Bangash, MN; Pareek, N; Pan, D; Sze, S; Minhas, JS; Hanif, W; Khunti, K. Ethnicity and COVID-19: An urgent public health research priority. *Lancet*, 2020, 30922-3, 1-2.

[12] Wu, JT; Leung, K; Leung, GM. Nowcasting and forecasting the potential domestic and international spread of the 2019-nCoV outbreak originating in Wuhan, China: A modelling study. *Lancet*, 2020, 395, 689-697.

[13] Horton. R. Offline: COVID-19 and the NHS—*A national scandal. Lancet*, 2020, 395, 1022-1022.

[14] Zhang, YZ; Koopmans, M; Yuen, KY; Andersen, K; Perlman, S; Hogue, B; Eckerle, I. The novel coronavirus outbreak: What we know and what we don't. *Cell*, 2020, 180, 1034-1036.

[15] The *Cell* Editorial Team. COVID-19: Navigating uncertainties together. *Cell*, 2020, 181, 209-210.

[16] Callaghan, S. COVID-19 is a data science issue. *Patterns*, 2020, 1, 100022–1-3.

[17] Liao, H; Zhang, L; Marley, G; Tang, W. Differentiating COVID-19 response strategies. *Innovation*, in press.

[18] Oberfeld, B; Achanta, A; Carpenter, K; Chen, P; Gilette, N; Langat, P; Said, J; Schiff, A; Zhou, A; Barczak, A; Pillai, S. COVID-19. *Cell*, in press.

[19] Blanco-Melo, D; Nilsson-Payant, BE; Liu, WC; Uhl, S; Hoagland, D; Møller, R; Jordan, TX; Oishi, K; Panis, M; Sachs, D; Wang, TT; Schwartz, RE; Lim, JK; Albrecht, RA; tenOever, B. R. Imbalanced host response to SARS-CoV-2 drives development of COVID-19. *Cell*, in press.

[20] Hoffmann, M; Kleine-Weber, H; Pöhlmann, S. A multibasic cleavage site in the spike protein of SARS-CoV-2 is essential for infection of human lung cells. *Mol. Cell*, in press.

[21] Ziegler, CGK; Allon, SJ; Nyquist, SK; Mbano, IM; Miao, VN; Tzouanas, CN; Cao, Y; Yousif, AS; Bals, J; Hauser, BM; Feldman, J; Muus, C; Wadsworth II, MH; Kazer, SW; Hughes, TK; Doran, B; Gatter, GJ; Vukovic, M; Taliaferro, F; Mead, BE; Guo, Z; Wang, JP; Gras, D; Plaisant, M; Ansari, M; Angelidis, I; Adler, H; Sucre, JMS; Taylor, CJ; Lin, B; Waghray, A; Mitsialis, V; Dwyer, DF; Buchheit, KM; Boyce, JA; Barrett, NA; Laidlaw, TM; Carroll, SL; Colonna, L; Tkachev, V; Peterson, CW; Yu, A; Zheng, HB; Gideon, HP; Winchell, CG; Lin, PL; Bingle, CD; Snapper, SB; Kropski, JA; Theis, FJ; Schiller, HB; Zaragosi, LE; Barbry, P; Leslie, A; Kiem, HP; Flynn, JL; Fortune, SM; Berger, B; Finberg, RW; Kean, LS; Garber, M; Schmidt, AG; Lingwood, D; Shalek, AK; Ordovas-Montanes, J. HCA Lung Biological Network. SARS-CoV-2 receptor ACE2 is an interferon-stimulated gene in human airway epithelial cells and is detected in specific cell subsets across tissues. *Cell*, in press.

[22] Paraskevis, D; Kostaki, EG; Magiorkinis, G; Panayiotakopoulos, G; Sourvinos, G; Tsiodras, S. Full-genome evolutionary analysis of the novel corona virus (2019-nCoV) rejects the hypothesis of emergence as a result of a recent recombination event. *Infect. Genet. Evol.*, 2020, 79, 104212–1-4.

[23] Chen, J. Pathogenicity and transmissibility of 2019-nCoV—A quick overview and comparison with other emerging viruses. *Microb. Infect.*, 2020, 22, 69-71.

[24] Lai, CC; Shih, TP; Ko, WC; Tang, HJ; Hsueh, PR. Severe acute respiratory syndrome coronavirus 2 (SARS-CoV-2) and coronavirus disease-2019 (COVID-19): The epidemic and the challenges. *Int. J. Antimicrob. Agents*, 2020, 55, 105924–1-9.

[25] Ashour, HM; Elkhatib, WF; Rahman, M; Elshabrawy, HA. Insights into the recent 2019 novel coronavirus (SARS-CoV-2) in light of past human coronavirus outbreaks. *Pathogens*, 2020, 9, 186–1-15.

[26] Xie, M; Chen, Q. Insight into 2019 novel coronavirus — An updated interim review and lessons from SARS-CoV and MERS-CoV. *Int. J. Infect. Dis.*, 2020, 94, 119-124.

[27] Peckham, H; de Gruijter, NM; Raine, C; Radziszewska, A; Ciurtin, C; Wedderburn, LR; Rosser, EC; Deakin, CT; Webb, K. Sex-bias in COVID-19: A meta-analysis and review of sex differences in disease and immunity. *Lancet Infect. Dis.* submitted for publication.

[28] Li, Y; Liu, B; Cui, J; Wang, Z; Shen, Y; Xu, Y; Yao, K; Guan, Y. *COVID-19 evolves in human hosts*, Xidian University–Peking University–University of Illinois at Chicago–University of Michigan, Working Paper, 2020, 1-24.

[29] Fuster, V; Turco, JV. COVID-19: A lesson in humility and an opportunity for sagacity and hope. *J. Am. Coll. Cardiol.*, in press.

[30] Yong, C. COVID-19: The isolation that has brought us together. *J. Am. Coll. Cardiol.*, in press.

[31] Thorlund, K; Dron, L; Park, J; Hsu, G; Forrest, JI; Mills, EJ. A real-time dashboard of clinical trials for COVID-19. *Lancet Dig. Health*, 2020, 30086-8–1-2.

[32] Hirano, T; Masaaki Murakami, M. COVID-19: A new virus, but a familiar receptor and cytokine release syndrome. *Immunity*, in press.

[33] Guo, D; Li, KC; Peters, TR; Snively, BM; Poehling, KA; Zhou, X. Multi-scale modeling for the transmission of influenza and the evaluation of interventions toward it. *Sci. Rep.*, 2015, 5, 8980–1-9.

[34] Arora, N; Schuenemann, VJ; Jäger, G; Peltzer, A; Seitz, A; Herbig, A; Strouhal, M; Grillová, L; Sánchez-Busó, L; Kühnert, D; Bos, KI; Rivero Davis, L; Mikalová, L; Bruisten, S; Komericki, P; French, P; Grant, PR; Pando, MA; Gallo Vaulet, L; Rodríguez Fermepin, M; Martinez, A; Centurion Lara, A; Giacani, L; Norris, SJ; Smajs, D; Bosshard, PP; González-Candelas, F; Nieselt, K; Krause, J; Bagheri, HC. Origin of modern syphilis and emergence of a pandemic *Treponema pallidum* cluster. *Nat. Microbiol.*, 2017, 2, 16245–1-6.

[35] Patiño-Galindo JÁ; Torres-Puente, M; Bracho, MA; Alastrué, I; Juan, A; Navarro, D; Galindo, MJ; Ocete, D; Ortega, E; Gimeno, C; Belda, J; Domínguez, V; Moreno, R; González-Candelas, F. The molecular epidemiology of HIV-1 in the Comunidad Valenciana (Spain): Analysis of transmission clusters. *Sci. Rep.*, 2017, 7, 11584–1-10.

[36] Patiño-Galindo, JÁ; González-Candelas, F; Pybus, OG. The effect of RNA substitution models on viroid and RNA virus phylogenies. *Genome Biol. Evol.*, 2018, 10, 657-666.

[37] De Wilde, AH; Snijder, EJ; Kikkert, M; van Hemert, MJ. Host factors in coronavirus replication. *Curr. Top. Microbiol. Immunol.*, 2018, 419, 1-42.

[38] Paules, CI; Marston, HD; Fauci, AS. Coronavirus infections—More than just the common cold. *J. Am. Med. Assoc.*, 2020, 323, 707-708.

[39] Kucharski, AJ; Kama, M; Watson, CH; Aubry, M; Funk, S; Henderson, AD; Brady, OJ; Vanhomwegen, J; Manuguerra, JC; Lau, CL; Edmunds, WJ; Aaskov, J; Nilles, EJ; Cao-Lormeau, VM; Hué, S; Hibberd, ML. Using paired serology and surveillance data to quantify dengue transmission and control during a large outbreak in Fiji. *eLife*, 2018, 7, e34848–1-26.

[40] Kucharski, A. *The Rules of Contagion: Why Things Spread — and Why They Stop*; Profile: London, UK, 2020.

[41] Wenham, C. Modelling can only tell us so much: Politics explains the rest. *Lancet*, 2020, 395, 1335-1335.

[42] Erlinger, TP. *Complexities of epidemics*, Resource 1, The American Institute of Dental Public Health: San Antonio, TX, 2020.

[43] Quevedo, L. personal communication.

In: COVID-19 Pandemic
Editor: A. K. Haghi
ISBN: 978-1-53618-565-2

Chapter 4

OLDER PEOPLE AND BCG VACCINE PROTECTION FROM SEVERE COVID-19

***Francisco Torrens*[1,*] *and Gloria Castellano*[2]**
[1]Institut Universitari de Ciència Molecular, Universitat de València, Edifici d'Instituts de Paterna, València, Spain
[2]Departamento de Ciencias Experimentales y Matemáticas, Facultad de Veterinaria y Ciencias Experimentales, Universidad Católica de Valencia San Vicente Mártir, València, Spain

ABSTRACT

The association between the coronavirus-disease-2019 pandemic and artificial intelligence results inspiring. Artificial intelligence presents many applications in diagnosis, therapeutics, epidemiology and public health in this coronavirus pandemic. *These smartphone data might result at the focus*. The doctor is the best placebo and the chair is the best diagnosis. The doctor should place the information in the processor; however, he should observe the sufferer's expression. Persons acquire the next messages from the coronavirus disease 2019 pandemic. Negative messages: (a) persons result totally susceptible not only as persons but as

* Corresponding Author's E-mail: torrens@uv.es.

a civilization; (b) they should be additionally careful as a civilization; (c) the socioeconomic influence results heading for putting them denoted. In optimistic messages, certain features result heading for altering civilization: (a) tele-labour; (b) distant help; (c) automatic sufferer discovery techniques.

Keywords: BCG vaccination policy, COVID-19 coronavirus, cross-protection, mortality, pandemic, artificial intelligence, ageing

1. Introduction

Setting the scene: coronavirus (CoV) disease 2019 (COVID-19), artificial intelligence (AI), older people before COVID-19 and bacillus Calmette-Guérin (BCG) vaccine protection from severe COVID-19. The relationship between COVID-19 pandemic and AI is stimulating. The AI has a lot of applications in diagnosis, therapeutics, epidemiology and public health (PH) in COVID-19 pandemic. The pandemic affects 217 countries and territories, with 12 000 000 infected subjects, 600 000 deaths and 7 000 000 recovered patients. A question (Q) was raised.

Q1. (M. González de Vega). What do you miss about confinement?

Galvez et al., informed in *Nereis* drugs repurposing for CoV treatment and computational study based on molecular topology [1]. Earlier publications reviewed COVID-19, hydroxychloroquine, drug repurposing, mathematics [2], PH, communication, history, COVID-19-pandemic challenge [3], flu, syphilis, human immunodeficiency virus, hepatitis, virus evolution, CoV and dengue [4].

The purpose of the present report is to review COVID-19, AI, older people before COVID-19 and BCG vaccine protection from severe COVID-19. The aim of this work is to initiate a debate by suggesting a number of questions (Q), which can arise when addressing subjects of what AI could take advantage of. It was provided, when possible, answers (A) and hypotheses (H) on the best placebo being the physician, the best diagnosis being the chair and the physician must put the data in the computer but he must look at the patient's face.

2. Older People before COVID-19

Redón Mas and Ariño Villarroya proposed Q/A/H on older people before COVID-19 [5].

Q1. (Ariño Villarroya). What could AI take advantage of?

A1. (Redón Mas). Situation: uncertainty and fear; people are faced with something unknown.

Q2. (Ariño Villarroya). Improvisation in protection equipment?

A2. (Redón Mas). Yes, but the professionalism of the staff has solved those difficulties.

Q3. (Ariño Villarroya). Appreciation, applause at 20:00?

A3. (Redón). It revealed the seams of health system (HS): financing; not to consider sanitary model.

Q4. (Ariño Villarroya). In addition, are people not thinking about the conditions for this change?

Q5. (Ariño Villarroya). Any important sewing for the transition from acute to chronic?

A5. (Redón). Budget; but structure must be changed for population sociodemographic structure.

Q6. (Ariño Villarroya). Difficulty understanding the development of the virus?

A6. (Redón Mas). There is no parallel: There are over 44 000 articles on COVID.

Q7. (Ariño). Severe acute respiratory syndrome (SARS)-CoV clade 2 (-2) is not a respiratory but a complex disease: when it affects, is it individualized?

A7. (Redón). Yes, whether or not it is capable of triggering the inflammatory storm varies greatly.

Q8. (Redón Mas). Who is going to go wrong or right?

Q9. (Redón Mas). What happens next?

A9. (Redón Mas). Complex response or pulmonary fibrosis, depression, delirium, etc.

Q10. (Ariño Villarroya). Sociodemographic and clinical risk factors (RFs)?

Q11. (Ariño Villarroya). Sex: are more women infected but more men die?

A11. (Redón Mas). Yes, but in all diseases.

Q12. (Redón Mas). Why?

A12. (Redón Mas). Not known.

Q13. (Ariño Villarroya). Is age key?

A13. (Redón Mas). Disease of which people knew little; the problem with age is comorbidities.

Q14. (Ariño Villarroya). The ethnic group?

A14. (Redón Mas). There are the socioeconomic aspects: the social level is an RF (in all diseases).

Q15. (Ariño). Immigrants in the picking of the pear in unacceptable living conditions are a key RF?

A15. (Redón Mas). Exactly.

Q16. (Ariño Villarroya). Diabetes?

A16. (Redón). Comorbidity; furthermore, with the inflammatory storm, vascular occlusion occurs.

Q17. (Ariño Villarroya). Is the blood system severely affected?

A17. (Redón Mas). Yes, there is vascular occlusion with thrombus production.

Q18. (Ariño Villarroya). Severe asthma?

A18. (Redón). Because bronchial tree is more loaded: asthma/chronic obstructive pulmonary disease.

Q19. (Ariño Villarroya). Cancer?

A19. (Redón Mas). It depends: in treatment (more risk); in complete remission (less risk).

Q20. (Ariño). The role of AI in helping us to overcome what was already possible and the future?

Q21. (Ariño Villarroya). In what aspects can AI be used and how can it be used, e.g., sentinel?

A21. (Redón). Jan. 10, 2020: a Canadian company warned that an infectious disease will spread from Wuhan.

Q22. (Ariño Villarroya). The sentinel system worked, but the alerts were ignored?

A22. (Redón). Predictive models were discontinued due to a lack of reliable data/previous models.

Q23. (Redón Mas). With all this information, how do people act?

Q24. (Redón Mas). Is it against individual liberties?

Q25. (Ariño Villarroya). In Spain, have people seen the chaos of the data?

A25. (Redón). People have 17 HSs, Ministry of Health had no structure and HS effectiveness fell.

Q26. (Ariño Villarroya). Are people information systems not up to par?

A26. (Redón). Problem is that systems do not talk to each other because they are different software.

Q27. (Ariño Villarroya). AI in therapies?

A27. (Redón). Possibility of studying the virus structures, therapeutic targets, activities, etc. existed.

Q28. (Redón Mas). The uncertainty was: what treatment do physicians give?

Q29. (Ariño Villarroya). What has been the path regarding treatment?

A29. (Redón). Remdesivir, hydroxychloroquine, dexamethasone and high-dose corticosteroids, etc.

Q30. (Ariño Villarroya). The obstacles to this AI?

A30. (Redón). Information-uniformity lack: common language; objective is that information be collected in real time.

Q31. (Ariño Villarroya). Is it purely technological or political?

A31. (Redón Mas). It exists, but it is worth money.

Q32. (Ariño Villarroya). Political interference?

A32. (Redón Mas). The concept that *this iphone information may be at the centre* is not assumed.

H1. (Redón Mas). The best placebo is the physician and the best diagnosis is the chair.

H2. (Redón). The physician must put the data in the computer but he must look at the patient's face.

Q33. (Ariño Villarroya). The percentage of anti-vaccines that would impede herd immunity?

A33. (Redón Mas). People know neither the immune capacity nor the capacity of vaccinations.

Q34. (Ariño Villarroya). Will the behaviour of this virus resemble others in its seasonal nature?

A34. (Redón Mas). It seems that there is no clear seasonal character.

Q35. (Ariño). It is a strange/unique virus: A part of the population does not understand precautions?

A35. (Redón). Air transmission exists; droplets are placed around the patient, who distributes them.

Q36. (Ariño Villarroya). What lessons have we learned?

A36. (Redón Mas). Bad: we are completely vulnerable not only as individuals but as a society; we must be more cautious as a society; the socioeconomic impact is going to leave us marked. Positive: telework; remote assistance; automated patient detection methods.

Q37. (Ariño Villarroya). In addition, in that area, do you think we also need a change in ethics?

A37. (Redón Mas). Yes, but when the vaccine come, these changes will go back a long way.

Q38. (Ariño Villarroya). Do not you think that even in AI itself people need another ethic?

A38. (Redón Mas). Yes, ethical thinking and attitudes are going to have to conform.

3. BCG Vaccine Protection from Severe Coronavirus Disease 2019 (COVID-19)

A series of epidemiological explorations suggested a negative association between national BCG vaccination policy, and COVID-19 prevalence and mortality. However, the comparisons are difficult to validate because of broad differences between countries (e.g., socioeconomic status, demographic structure, rural *vs*. urban settings, time of arrival of the pandemic, number of diagnostic tests, criteria for testing) and national control strategies to limit COVID-19 spread. Evidence for a potential biobasis of BCG cross-protection from severe COVID-19 was reviewed, and the epidemiological analysis was refined to mitigate effects of potentially confounding factors (e.g., COVID-19-epidemic stage, development, rurality, population density, age structure) [6]. A correlation between BCG index, an estimation of the degree of universal BCG vaccination deployment in a country, and COVID-19 mortality in different socially similar European countries was observed, indicating that every 10% rise in BCG index was associated with a 10.4% decay in COVID-19 mortality. Results fail to confirm the null hypothesis of no association between BCG vaccination and COVID-19 mortality, and suggest that BCG could present a protective effect. Nevertheless, the analyses are restricted to coarse-scale signals and must be considered with caution. Clinical trials of BCG vaccination are required to corroborate the detected patterns, and to establish causality between BCG vaccination and protection from severe COVID-19. Implications of PH of a plausible BCG cross-protection from severe COVID-19 are discussed.

4. Final Remarks

From the present results and discussion, the following final remarks can be drawn.

1. This iphone information may be at the centre.
2. The best placebo is the physician and the best diagnosis is the chair.
3. The physician must put the data in the computer but he must look at the patient's face.
4. People have learned the following lessons from the coronavirus disease 2019 pandemic. Bad points: (a) people are completely vulnerable not only as individuals but as a society; (b) they must be more cautious as a society; (c) the socioeconomic impact is going to leave them marked. In positive points, the following aspects are going to transform society: (a) telework; (b) remote assistance; (c) automated patient detection methods.

ACKNOWLEDGMENTS

The authors acknowledge Dr. Vicente Simón by the online courses *Mindfulness in Times of Crisis* and financial support from Fundación Universidad Católica de Valencia *San Vicente Mártir* (Project No. 2019-217-001UCV).

REFERENCES

[1] Galvez, J., Zanni, R., Galvez-Llompart, M. Drugs repurposing for coronavirus treatment: Computational study based on molecular topology. *Nereis* 2020, 2020(12), 15-18.

[2] Torrens, F., Castellano, G. COVID-19, hydroxychloroquine, drug repurposing and mathematics. In: *COVID-19 Pandemic: Questions, Answers and Hypotheses*; Haghi, A. K. (Ed.); Nova: Hauppauge, NY, in press.

[3] Torrens, F., Castellano, G. Public health, communication, history, COVID-19-pandemic challenge. In *COVID-19 Pandemic: Questions, Answers and Hypotheses*; Haghi, A. K., (Ed.); Nova: Hauppauge, NY, in press.

[4] Torrens, F., Castellano, G. Flu, syphilis, HIV, hepatitis, virus evolution, coronavirus and dengue. In *COVID-19 Pandemic: Questions, Answers and Hypotheses*, Haghi, A. K., (Ed.); Nova: Hauppauge, NY, in press.

[5] Redón Mas, J., Ariño Villarroya, A., personal communication.

[6] Escobar, L. E., Molina-Cruz, A., Barillas-Mury, C. BCG vaccine protection from severe coronavirus disease 2019 (COVID-19). *Proc. Natl. Acad. Sci. U. S. A.* 2020, 2008410117-1-7.

In: COVID-19 Pandemic
Editor: A. K. Haghi
ISBN: 978-1-53618-565-2

Chapter 5

CoV, Illusion, Gastrointestinal System, Remdesivir, Confinement, Youth

Francisco Torrens[1,*] and Gloria Castellano[2]
[1]Institut Universitari de Ciència Molecular, Universitat de València, Edifici d'Instituts de Paterna, València, Spain
[2]Departamento de Ciencias Experimentales y Matemáticas, Facultad de Veterinaria y Ciencias Experimentales, Universidad Católica de Valencia San Vicente Mártir, València, Spain

Abstract

This review refers to the *grouting* of glances in relation to a subject. A bit in the style of a *new age* self-help book, this revision seeks to turn to the experts, as if they were a spiritual master capable of illuminating the path that helps people out of the dark cavern, in which they suddenly realized they were always secluded. For all the mysteries surrounding coronavirus disease 2019, one thing is certain: People cannot be lulled into a false sense of security. Surely it results not that the virus is now

* Corresponding Author's E-mail: torrens@uv.es.

less aggressive, but that people are more vigilant. Once people determined which bacteria are associated with coronavirus severity, they could design treatments or diets to modify them. The scientific community, and the health and regulatory authorities, must monitor all the clinical data that will be provided to confirm definitively the suitability of remdesivir treatment. A study will allow analysing how the measures adopted by each government affected. One can identify elements of the collective security system as the foundation for directing action. A decalogue for reflection was proposed towards a non-classroom university. People must devise ways to regain normality without putting the lives of their population at risk.

Keywords: pandemic, pathogen, coronavirus, virus, infection, 2019-nCoV, COVID-19

1. Introduction

Setting the scene: how the coronavirus (CoV) escapes an evolutionary trade-off that helps keep other pathogens in check, if severe acute respiratory syndrome (SARS)-CoV clade 2 (-2) has lost aggressiveness, bewaring of deceptive viral illusions, the bacteria of people's gastrointestinal system (GIS), allies against CoV disease 2019 (COVID-19), what remdesivir, the first authorized drug against COVID-19 that Trump wants to capture, is, if confinement leaves people with consequences, what the responses to COVID-19 and violent extremism have in common, the emotional and behavioural consequences of confinement, young people with open faces, how to encourage them to protect themselves from CoV, towards a non-classroom university, decalogue for essential reflection, why the World Health Organisation (WHO) say the worst is yet to come, journalism in the COVID-19 era as a compliment to the treatment of sources, COVID-19 outbreaks being inevitable but could protect people from a second wave, COVID-19 and people being a long way from group immunity.

The pandemic affects 217 countries and territories, with 13 000 000 infected subjects, 600 000 deaths and 7 000 000 recovered patients. A question (Q) was raised on journalism in COVID-19 era.

Q1. (Eva Herrero). How can we achieve rigor in journalism?

Galvez et al., informed in *Nereis* drugs repurposing for CoV treatment and computational study based on molecular topology [1]. Earlier publications reviewed COVID-19, hydroxychloroquine, drug repurposing, mathematics [2], public health, communication, history, COVID-19-pandemic challenge [3], flu, syphilis, human immunodeficiency virus, hepatitis, virus evolution, CoV, dengue [4], older people and bacillus Calmette-Guérin (BCG) vaccine protection from severe COVID-19 [5].

The purpose of the present report is to review how CoV escapes an evolutionary trade-off that helps keep other pathogens in check, if SARS-CoV-2 has lost aggressiveness, bewaring of deceptive viral illusions, the bacteria of people's GIS, allies against COVID-19, what remdesivir, the first authorized drug against COVID-19 that Trump wants to capture, is, if confinement leaves people with consequences, what the responses to COVID-19 and violent extremism have in common, the emotional and behavioural consequences of confinement, young people with open faces, how to encourage them to protect themselves from CoV, towards a non-classroom university and decalogue for essential reflection, why the WHO say the worst is yet to come, journalism in the COVID-19 era as a compliment to the treatment of sources, COVID-19 outbreaks being inevitable but could protect people from a second wave, COVID-19 and people being a long way from group immunity.

2. How CoV Escapes a Trade-Off that Helps Keep Other Pathogens in Check

Viruses walk a fine line between severity and transmissibility [6]. If they are too virulent, they kill or incapacitate their hosts: *This limits their ability to infect* new hosts [7]. Conversely, viruses that cause little harm may not be *generating enough copies of themselves* to be infectious. For all the mysteries surrounding COVID-19, one thing is certain: People cannot be lulled into a false sense of security. As Sun Tzu warned in *The Art of War*, know your enemy. A great deal more to know about SARS-CoV-2 exists before people claim any victories.

3. Has SARS-CoV-2 Lost Aggressiveness? Beware of Viral Illusions

Surely it results not that the virus is now less aggressive, but that people are more vigilant [8]. It results people's train that started to move and not the one next door. However, people must be cautious and patient to avoid falling into viral illusions.

4. The Bacteria of Our Gastrointestinal System, Allies vs. COVID-19

Once people determined which bacteria are associated with COVID-19 severity, they could design treatments or diets to modify them in a matter of days [9]. It may be possible to reduce the inflammatory response modifying the intestinal biota to protect people from the more serious COVID-19 consequences. Increasing bacterial diversity, people protect themselves not only from viral infections, but also vs. other health problems, e.g., mental health.

5. What is Remdesivir, the First Authorized Drug Against COVID-19

The scientific community, together with the health and regulatory authorities, must closely monitor all the clinical data that will be provided in the coming months to confirm definitively the suitability of remdesivir treatment [10].

6. Does Confinement Leave People with Consequences?

A study will allow analysing how the measures adopted by each government or public administration affected [11]. However, the impact of the sociocultural differences of each country on the ability of people to adapt and face the current situation. Two aspects to prevent similar situations in future pandemics.

7. What do COVID-19 Responses and Violent Extremism Have in Common?

Despite the differences, one can identify elements of the collective security system as the foundation for directing action *vs.* the pandemic [12]: the need to direct the response to the safety of all its members; special protection must be given to the weakest or most vulnerable in the quest for collective security; the answer must be based on cooperative relationships. Perhaps, it is a model that works again, this time in the fight *vs.* another virus: that of the spread of extremist ideas that polarize societies and justify violence *vs.* the other. Without a doubt, the response to the next viral wave will be easier if people managed to analyze the situation and the response in cooperative and collective security terms.

8. The Emotional and Behavioural Consequences of Confinement

As people have clearer information about the survival of the virus on different surfaces, possible treatments or the vaccine, people will be more tolerant of the potential risk of contagion [13].

9. Young People with Open Faces: How to Encourage Them to Protect?

People can encourage others to protect themselves and their environment [14]: knowing that the place from where something is heard is more important than the content of what is said; the contents must aim not at the regulations but at producing effects of liability linked to others (friends, family) for which their actions could have serious consequences; to make social and media visible (*influencers via*) the serious effects that COVID-19 *has among some young people*. When the above fails (because people know that not everything is educable and that not everyone agrees to give up their satisfaction) sanctions and vigilance exist. Their irresponsibility, unlike those who justify it with their cynicism, is a false temporary exit.

10. Towards a Non-Classroom University? Decalogue for Reflection

Some ideas and approaches on a non-classroom university follow [15]: (1) the advance of *online* is so evident and unstoppable that it does not deserve any discussion; (2) one must try to avoid the risk of succumbing to false dilemmas between face-to-face and *online*, and flee from exclusive positions that place people at one of the extremes, without exploring the *hybrid* territory in which both must necessarily meet; (3) it is educated by contagion (it is not necessary to flee from the virus) and, therefore, the environment and the places of contact and relationship are essential in the training process; (4) new technologies offer enormous opportunities for educational renewal; (5) the supports are essential, but people must know what to do with them; (6) teachers will always remain the basic piece and the decisive element of the training process, which can never be dispensed with and for which an environment and conditions are required to guarantee their accessibility, presence and proximity; (7) but the teacher's roles and functions must be redefined, to combine simultaneously the role of teacher, guide, prescriber, companion, inspirer and even *influencer*; (8) this entails greater dedication and new tasks for that *weak link* in the chain that is usually teachers, and confronts them with new tasks and more extensive, diverse and complex tasks, which require additional efforts and undoubtedly require better organization and wide endowment of resources; (9) perhaps now more popular than ever is this popular claim that *knowledge has no place*; (10) *online*, and digital methods and supports constitute an element of indisputable and enormous potential for teaching, particularly for the advancement of personalized programs supported by instruments (e.g., *big data*, artificial intelligence).

11. Why does the WHO Say the Worst is Yet to Come?

The worst is yet to come [16]. Apparently, a prophecy that perhaps does not require great prophets. However, the phrase was not so much the prediction of an inescapable future as a call to work to avoid or, at least, reduce that *worst*. An appeal not to let down people's guard and to make even greater efforts to control the pandemic. The worst is yet to come, but it can be much *less worse* with effort and solidarity. Much less worse the less people be.

12. Journalism in COVID-19 Era: A Compliment to the Treatment of Sources

During the months of health alarm, journalists have not stopped searching for stories, contrasting them and verifying them [17]. People have all witnessed a more rigorous journalism where testimonies and sources helped differentiate information from disinformation. A well-informed society is a freer, fairer, more democratic society, more committed to its community and above all with critical thinking that will advance it to the future of well-being [18].

13. Covid Outbreaks Are Inevitable But Could Protect from a Second Wave

Given that it is not positive to maintain confinement indefinitely, people must devise ways to regain normality without putting the lives of their most vulnerable population at risk [19]. It is worth highlighting measures to achieve the balance: (1) to strengthen health systems, with special attention to medical care services for the elderly in homes and nursing homes; (2) to devise rapid diagnostic tests, if possible in saliva, cheap and for sale in pharmacies, that could be repeated as many times as convenient, to isolate quickly the positive cases and find out who is immunized; (3) it is essential to reaffirm the social distancing measures in coexistence (masks, avoiding physical contact, frequent hand cleaning, activities in open spaces, etc.) especially with the elderly.

14. COVID-19: People Are a Long Way from Group Immunity

Ultimately, the only way to escape truly COVID-19 pandemic is to achieve group immunity on a large scale, everywhere, not just in a small number of places where infections were highest [20]. Meanwhile, uncertainty about the naturally acquired threshold to prevent the spread of the virus and reduce the R_0 value as much as possible only leaves one way to go: distancing, facemasking, testing and contact tracing everywhere. Therefore, calm and patience.

15. Final Remarks

From the present results and discussion, the following final remarks can be drawn.

1. For all the mysteries surrounding coronavirus disease 2019, one thing is certain: People cannot be lulled into a false sense of security. As Sun Tzu warned in *The Art of War*, know your enemy. A great deal more to know about severe acute respiratory syndrome coronavirus clade 2 exists before people claim any victories.
2. Surely it results not that the virus is now less aggressive, but that people are more vigilant. It results people's train that started to move and not the one next door. However, people must be cautious and patient to avoid falling into viral illusions.
3. Once people determined which bacteria are associated with coronavirus severity, they could design treatments or diets to modify them. It may be possible to reduce the inflammatory response modifying the intestinal biota to protect people from the coronavirus consequences.
4. The scientific community, together with the health and regulatory authorities, must closely monitor all the clinical data that will be provided in the coming months to confirm definitively the suitability of remdesivir treatment.
5. A study will allow analysing how the measures adopted by each government or public administration affected. However, the impact

of the sociocultural differences of each country on the ability of people to adapt and face the current situation.

6. Despite the differences, one can identify elements of the collective security system as the foundation for directing action *vs.* the pandemic: the need to direct the response to the safety of all its members; special protection must be given to the weakest or most vulnerable in the quest for collective security; the answer must be based on cooperative relationships.
7. A decalogue for reflection was proposed towards a non-classroom university. Given that it is not positive to maintain confinement indefinitely, people must devise ways to regain normality without putting the lives of their most vulnerable population at risk.

Acknowledgments

The authors acknowledge Dr. Vicente Simón by the online courses *Mindfulness in Times of Crisis* and financial support from Fundación Universidad Católica de Valencia *San Vicente Mártir* (Project No. 2019-217-001UCV).

References

[1] Galvez, J., Zanni, R., Galvez-Llompart, M. Drugs repurposing for coronavirus treatment: Computational study based on molecular topology. *Nereis* 2020, 2020 (12), 15-18.

[2] Torrens, F., Castellano, G. COVID-19, hydroxychloroquine, drug repurposing and mathematics. In: *COVID-19 Pandemic: Questions, Answers and Hypotheses*; Haghi, A. K. (Ed.); Nova: Hauppauge, NY, in press.

[3] Torrens, F., Castellano, G. Public health, communication, history, COVID-19-pandemic challenge. In *COVID-19 Pandemic: Questions,*

Answers and Hypotheses; Haghi, A. K., (Ed.); Nova: Hauppauge, NY, in press.

[4] Torrens, F., Castellano, G. Flu, syphilis, HIV, hepatitis, virus evolution, coronavirus and dengue. In *COVID-19 Pandemic: Questions, Answers and Hypotheses*, Haghi, A. K., (Ed.); Nova: Hauppauge, NY, in press.

[5] Torrens, F., Castellano, G. Older people and BCG vaccine protection from severe COVID-19. In *COVID-19 Pandemic: Questions, Answers and Hypotheses*, Haghi, A. K., (Ed.); Nova: Hauppauge, NY, in press.

[6] Aktipis, A., Alcock, J. How the coronavirus escapes an evolutionary trade-off that helps keep other pathogens in check. *Conversation* 2020, 2020 (Jun. 17), 1-1.

[7] Aktipis, A., Alcock, J. El coronavirus se comporta como una enfermedad de transmisión sexual. *Conversation* 2020, 2020 (Jun. 23), 1-1. [The coronavirus behaves like a sexually transmitted disease.]

[8] Pita, M. ¿Ha perdido agresividad el SARS-CoV-2? Cuidado con las ilusiones víricas engañosas. *Conversation* 2020, 2020 (Jun. 27), 1-1. [Has SARS-CoV-2 lost its aggressiveness? Beware of deceptive viral illusions]

[9] Villapol, S. Las bacterias de nuestro sistema gastrointestinal, aliadas contra la COVID-19. *Conversation* 2020, 2020 (Jul. 1), 1-1. [Bacteria in our gastrointestinal system, allied against COVID-19]

[10] López-Muñoz, F., Guerra Guirao, J. A. Qué es el remdesivir, el primer fármaco autorizado contra la COVID-19 que Trump quiere acaparar. *Conversation* 2020, 2020 (Jul. 1), 1-1. [What is remdesivir, the first authorized drug against COVID-19 that Trump wants to monopolize]

[11] López Fernández, D., Sanz, A. ¿Nos deja secuelas el confinamiento? *Conversation* 2020, 2020 (Jul. 1), 1-1. [Does confinement leave us sequels?]

[12] Bermejo, R. ¿Qué tienen en común las respuestas a la COVID-19 y al extremismo violento? *Conversation* 2020, 2020 (Jul. 2), 1-1. [What do responses to COVID-19 and violent extremism have in common?]

[13] Luis, E. Las consecuencias emocionales y de comportamiento que nos deja el confinamiento. *Conversation* 2020, 2020 (Jul. 2), 1-1. [The emotional and behavioral consequences of confinement]

[14] Ubieto Pardo, J. R. Jóvenes a cara descubierta: ¿Cómo animarles a protegerse del coronavirus? *Conversation* 2020, 2020 (Jul. 5), 1-1. [Young people uncovered: How to encourage them to protect themselves from the coronavirus?]

[15] Vázquez, J. A. ¿Hacia una Universidad no presencial? Decálogo para una reflexión imprescindible. *Conversation* 2020, 2020 (Jul. 5), 1-1. [Towards a remote university? Decalogue for an essential reflection]

[16] Peiró, S. ¿Por qué dice la OMS que lo peor está por venir? *Conversation* 2020, 2020 (Jul. 6), 1-1. [Why does the WHO say that the worst is yet to come?]

[17] Herrero, E. Periodismo en la era de COVID-19, un elogio al tratamiento de las fuentes. *Telos* 2020, 2020 (Jul. 6), 1-1. [Journalism in the era of COVID-19, a compliment to the treatment of sources]

[18] Herrero, E. Periodismo en la era de COVID-19: Un elogio al tratamiento de las fuentes. *Conversation* 2020, 2020 (Jul. 6), 1-1. [Journalism in the Age of COVID-19: A Praise for the Treatment of Sources]

[19] Soriano, V. Los brotes de COVID-19 son inevitables, pero podrían protegernos de una segunda ola. *Conversation* 2020, 2020 (Jul. 7), 1-1. [COVID-19 outbreaks are inevitable, but could protect us from a second wave]

[20] Peinado Lorca, M., Monje, L. COVID-19: Estamos muy lejos de la inmunidad de grupo. *Conversation* 2020, 2020 (Jul. 8), 1-1. [We are a long way from group immunity.]

About the Editor

A. K. Haghi, PhD, is the author and editor of 165 books, as well as 1000 published papers in various journals and conference proceedings. Dr. Haghi has received several grants, consulted for a number of major corporations, and is a frequent speaker to national and international audiences. Since 1983, he served as professor at several universities. He is former Editor-in-Chief of the International Journal of Chemoinformatics and Chemical Engineering and Polymers Research Journal; and is on the editorial boards of many international journals. He is also a member of the Canadian Research and Development Center of Sciences and Cultures (CRDCSC), Montreal, Quebec, Canada. He holds a BSc in urban and environmental engineering from the University of North Carolina (USA), an MSc in mechanical engineering from North Carolina A&T State University (USA), a DEA in applied mechanics, acoustics and materials from the Université de Technologie de Compiègne (France), and a PhD in engineering sciences from Université de Franche-Comté (France).

INDEX

#

A

B

C

D

E

F

G

H

I

J

L

M

N

U

V

W

Y